HEALING

WITH

MAGNETS

HEALING
WITH
MAGNETS

GARY NULL, PH.D.

CARROLL & GRAF PUBLISHERS, INC.
NEW YORK

The author would like to acknowledge Patric Jennings for a super research effort, Lois Zinn for transcribing dozens of interviews, Vickie Riba Koestler for digital editing, and Vickie Hughs for tirelessly arranging the dozens of inter-views.

First Carroll & Graf edition 1998

Carroll & Graf Publishers, Inc.
19 West 21st Street
New York, NY 10010

Library of Congress Cataloging in Publication Data is available.

ISBN: 0-7867-0530-2

Manufactured in the United States of America

Contents

INTRODUCTION

The power of the magnet is one of the most basic powers in nature. We know that magnetism itself was an ingredient in the primordial soup from which the universe and our planet came forth. Magnetism is the force that keeps order in the galaxy, allowing stars and planets to spin at significant velocities. And in a sense, our own planet's magnetic field is responsible for protecting all life on earth.

This book is about how we can use the power of magnetism to optimize health. Today, we are at an exciting juncture in the evolution of health care as biomagnetic therapy fast becomes one of the most promising new therapeutic interventions. Actually, biomagnetic therapy is not new to everyone. Many veterinarians have been aware of biomagnetic benefits for years, and use magnets to heal fractures quickly, thereby saving the lives of racehorses and other animals. Doctors treating professional athletes commonly recommend magnets to speed up recovery from painful injuries. And other physicians in a variety of specialties, including dermatologists, internists, pediatricians, and surgeons, are seeing excellent results as well.

That magnetic healing is nothing new can be seen by looking at early records of scientifically advanced civilizations, which tell us that magnetic forces have long been prized for their restorative properties. Ancient Greece discovered the very first natural magnet in the form of the lodestone, and Hippocrates, the father of medicine, noted its healing powers. The Egyptians, too, described the divine powers of the magnet in their writings, and Cleopatra frequently adorned herself with magnetic jewelry to preserve her youthfulness. Chinese manuscripts dating back thousands of years describe the Eastern belief that the life force, termed *qi,* is generated by the earth's magnetic field. Today, many believe that certain places on earth, such as Lourdes, France, and Sedona, Arizona, owe their healing powers to naturally high levels of this qi, or biomagnetic energy.

It should be noted that today, magnetic therapy is well established in other countries, such as Japan, China, India, Austria, and Germany. In the United States, unfortunately, many healing techniques readily accepted by other traditions are only familiar to those practitioners on the cutting edge. Although state-of-the-art American medicine uses techniques to monitor magnetic fields, such as electrocardiograms, electroencephalograms, and magnetic resonance imaging, it has not taken other forms of magnetic therapy seriously. More and more American studies, however, are confirming the value of the magnetic approach. As a result, magnet therapy is gaining credibility in the United States and being applied by increasing numbers of doctors and other health practitioners to treat a wide range of ailments. Now awareness of this modality is filtering down to the general public, as increasing numbers of people are sleeping on magnetic beds at night and wearing small magnets during the day for greater energy, preventive purposes, and healing. It is with the idea of expanding this awareness of a natural healing option that I have interviewed a wide range of clinicians, scientists, and patients, and written this book.

Finally, no one claims that magnetic therapy is going to work for everyone. However, ample clinical and personal evidence suggests that people experience a beneficial effect. One is led to ponder whether when Hippocrates wrote, "The natural force within each of us is that greatest healer of all," he did not have magnetic energy in mind.

HEALING

WITH

MAGNETS

Issues in Magnet Therapy

Research into magnet therapy is divided into two distinct areas: pulsed bioelectric magnetic therapy and fixed magnetic therapy. Probably 85 to 90 percent of the scientific literature is on pulsed bioelectric biomagnetic therapy; the remainder is on therapy with fixed solid magnets. As is always the case, research interest and funding have been where there is proprietary gain. No patents can be issued for work done on fixed magnets, but certainly they can be for pulsed magnetic devices. Since it cannot necessarily be assumed that a positive result from pulsed bioelectric magnets will automatically translate to a positive result from a fixed magnet, there needs to be more study in the area of fixed magnets.

Another reality of this still developing field is that there are different schools of thought on the essential mechanisms of magnetic therapy, centered on questions of polarity, among other issues. In this book I have tried to draw on the input of the most responsible scientific and medical representatives from varying points of view. These are not lay marketeers passing along misinformation. Rather, these sources are qualified M.D., Ph.D. research scientists, and clinicians who have spent years in the field.

One is Dr. William Pawluk, of Chicago, a board-certified family physician in both Canada and the United States and Assistant Professor in the School of Hygiene and Public Health and School of Medicine at Johns Hopkins University. Dr. Pawluk, who is vice president of the North American Academy of Magnetic Therapy, lectures extensively on magnetism and combines magnetic therapy and acupuncture in his practice. He has written a chapter on magnetic therapy for the *Textbook of Complementary Medicine* (Williams & Wilkins, Baltimore) and has undertaken the noble task of studying and translating a comprehensive body of foreign research on magnetism and its applications.

Another perspective comes from John Zimmerman, Ph.D., one of the leading authorities in America on the subject of magnets. He is president of the Bio-Electro-Magnetics Institute, an independent nonprofit educational research organization dedicated to furthering our understanding of bioelectromagnetism. Dr. Zimmerman has published extensively and is currently conducting a double-blind, placebo-controlled study on the effectiveness of fixed magnets for lower back pain. He is also a member of the North American Academy of Magnetic Therapy.

On some points the two main schools of thought think alike. They generally agree in their discussion of size, strength, and placement of magnets, and duration of treatment. Where they disagree is at the basic physics level regarding when to use a positive or a negative pole. There is also some confusion, as we shall see, about the correct labeling of poles on magnets. But controversy is par for the course in a developing field, and irrespective of which school is ultimately found right, each has enough positive clinical, anecdotal, and scientific results to show that magnets work.

MAGNETISM AND ELECTROMAGNETISM

What is the difference between a fixed magnet and an electromagnetic device? Simply put, a fixed magnet emits a magnetic field, while an electromagnetic apparatus gives off an electric and magnetic field. Dr. John Zimmerman elaborates: "Magnetism and electromagnetism are different sides of the same coin. However, unlike a coin, electromagnetism has three sides rather than two. They are the electric field, the magnetic field, and the electromagnetic radiation.

"Electric fields are associated with the displacement of charged particles, usually electrons, but sometimes charged particles called ions. An example of an electric field occurs when you shuffle your feet across a carpet and touch a doorknob. The carpet pulls some electrons from your body and your clothing, leaving you with a deficiency and the carpet with an excess. When you touch the doorknob, it pulls up electrons to satisfy your deficiency, and it balances the electrical charge, creating a spark in the process. Electrical fields are measured in units called volts per meter (vpm) or volts per centimeter (vpc).

"The next side of the three-sided coin is the magnetic field. A magnetic field is caused by electrical charges in motion, as opposed to an electric field, which is produced by electrical charges in different concentrations, more in one place than the other, regardless of whether or not they are moving. You cannot see the electrical current in a magnet; you have to delve deeper into the structure of matter to understand.

"In a static magnet, the electrical current moves in terms of electrons orbiting around the atomic nuclei. An iron body is magnetized when the electrons become aligned to a greater degree."

Zimmerman goes on to explain that the best way to describe magnetism in a permanent magnet is to make an analogy with the military: "Imagine all the atoms in an unmagnetized block of iron to be soldiers in a barracks going about their daily business. Some may be brushing their teeth, while others read magazines, and others lie in bed. Then, the captain walks in, and the drill sergeant says, 'Fall in.' Everybody scrambles to fall in place, aligning themselves in the same direction with a certain amount of space between them. The difference before and after the command 'Fall in' is analogous to the difference between an unmagnetized block of iron before and after being subjected to a magnetizing force. The magnetizing force commands electrons, and the atoms in the block of material literally fall into place. Once they become aligned in the same direction, you have a permanent magnet."

Magnetism can also be produced by currents in a wire, Zimmerman continues, and these magnetic fields are due to the electrons in the wire. "If it's a 60 cycles per second (cps) current, like a wall outlet, electrons shuffle back and forth, creating 60 full cps. But they really don't go anywhere. They're like the tide going in and out of the ocean, going first in one direction and then the other. But the tide really never goes anywhere outside of that predetermined length of run. Electrons in a wire, in a lamp cord, or in a power line, are very similar. They'll basically go back and forth, producing a magnetic field in the area around it."

How does this differ from electromagnetic radiation? This is the third side of the coin, Zimmerman explains. "EMR occurs when you have charges that accelerate or decelerate very quickly. Imagine a glass of water filled almost to the very top. You slowly dip a spoon into and out of the water, and every time you change direction, you accelerate the motion of the spoon. If the rate of that acceleration and deceleration is relatively slow, you can dip the spoon in and out of the nearly full glass of water all day long, and not much will happen. The water will stick to the spoon, and when you pull the spoon out of the water, it will have some water droplets adhere to it. When you put it back in, it will go back into the glass of water.

"What happens, though, if you start to accelerate the motion of that spoon? Obviously, water is going to start flying off of it. This is exactly what happens when you produce EMR. At a certain rate of change of velocity that is analogous to moving a spoon into and out of the water very quickly, charged particles, called photons, come off of the source of the moving electric charges, much like water droplets coming off of the spoon that's rapidly moving in and out of the glass of water. Photons, noncharged massless entities which carry the electromagnetic force across space, are frequently pulled off of the charged couriers, much like water droplets coming off the spoon being rapidly lowered into and raised from a glass of water. This is what we refer to as EMR." As the name implies, electromagnetic radiation contains two distinct fields: an electric field, measured in volts per meter or volts per centimeter, and a magnetic field, which is measured in units called teslas, or gauss. (One tesla equals 10,000 gauss.)

The effectiveness of using pulsed magnetic fields to heal bone fractures and, to a lesser degree, soft-tissue injuries such as sprains and strains, is quite well documented. Numerous scientific journals have reported these findings since the 1970s, and the FDA approves the use of pulsed electromagnetic fields for the treatment of nonunion bone fractures, which are fractures that will not heal on their own. It is believed that the pulsed electromagnetic fields penetrate the cast and get to the layer of skin that's moist and conductive. Then the electric field stops, but the magnetic field continues to do the healing work.

Clinical experience suggests other uses for electromagnetic devices. Hundreds of articles substantiate claims of benefit for a large number of conditions, including osteoarthritis, rheumatoid arthritis, fibromyalgia, tension headaches, migraines, and Parkinson's disease.

Fixed magnets are believed to help these conditions, as well as others, and are generally more economical and less complicated to use. Doctors have presented papers at the North American Academy of Magnetic Therapy, citing success with fixed magnets in patients with congestive heart failure and various types of cancerous conditions. A Canadian research project is investigating the effects of fixed magnets on fibromyalgia; specifically, the researchers want to determine whether sleeping on a magnetic pad helps to reduce the pain associated with the condition. Rheumatoid and osteoarthritis have been reported to respond very well to magnetic field therapy using fixed individual magnets.

THE POLAR CONTROVERSIES

If you're looking for confusion, controversy, and contradictions, you might want to follow politics, or better yet, you might want to look into the questions surrounding the naming of magnetic poles. For instance, is the south pole true south? And is the north pole true north? How a magnetic pole is named is dependent upon convention, and not all conventions are alike. Therefore, you may be getting two magnets from two companies where corresponding sides are called north on one magnet and south on the other. Dr. Zimmerman explains: "We need to understand that there are two ways of naming the north pole of the magnet: convention one and convention two. You have to know which convention you're dealing with. Otherwise, what you're calling north, somebody else may be calling south.

"Way one of naming the poles of the magnet is called the traditional, scientific, sailor navigation type of way. It assumes that if you suspend a bar magnet on a pivot point, like a compass needle, or maybe on a string from the ceiling, the part of the magnet that points north is labeled the north pole of the magnet, and obviously that end of the magnet that points geographically south is the south pole of the magnet." Zimmerman says that this traditional way of naming the poles is not the one used by most people employing biomagnetic therapy.

"In the biomagnetic nomenclature of identifying the poles of the magnet, it's just the opposite," Zimmerman explains. "That end of the magnet that points north is labeled the south pole because it's attracted to the north pole of the earth. That end of the magnet that attracts the south pole of the earth is labeled the north pole of the magnet because opposites attract." The north pole is often times referred to as the negative pole; the south pole is called the positive side of a magnet.

Zimmerman goes on: "People might say, 'Gee, in the traditional way of naming magnets, how can the north pole be pointing north?' The answer uses rather complex reasoning. I don't mean to confuse people, but in the traditional way of naming the poles of the magnet, the reason the north pole of the magnet points north is that the traditionalists assume that the south magnetic pole of the earth is located in the northern hemisphere. That sounds backwards, complex, and confusing, and it is. But that's the way traditional science textbooks and physics textbooks often get around the conundrum that the north pole of the magnet is pointing north. They say that the south pole is located in the northern hemisphere.

"That's all very confusing to people, so we like to focus our attention on what we call the biomagnetic definition, which avoids that complexity. It assumes that the north pole of the magnet is where it's supposed to be—in the geographic north pole of the earth, and the south pole is in the southern hemisphere. With this definition, a suspended bar magnet, or the arrowhead of a compass needle that points north, is always the south end of the magnet or the south end of the compass needle. Stated another way, if you have a magnet that is flat, and you want to know which end is north, approach it with a compass needle. That end of the magnet that attracts the arrowhead of the compass needle is the biomagnetic north pole."

Another controversy revolves around the issue of when to use the north, or negative, pole and when to use the south, or positive. One school of thought is based on the ideas of Davis and Rawls, whose studies done in the 1930s suggest that exposure to biomagnetic negative poles enhance health, while biomagnetic positive poles exacerbate disease. More recently, Dr. William Philpott has been championing the Davis and Rawls point of view and drawing conclusions based upon his own clinical experience. Here is what Philpott feels each pole will do:

North (Negative) Pole

Relieves pain
Reduces swelling

Promotes tissue alkalinization
Promotes sound, restful sleep
Increases tissue oxygenation
Calms the nervous system
Assists in relief of addictive tendencies

South (Positive) Pole

Accelerates growth indiscriminately
Increases swelling
Promotes tissue acidity
Decreases tissue oxygenation
Makes sleep less sound and restful
Promotes anxiety

There are those who support the claims of Philpott. Yet, scientists wishing to duplicate the work of Davis and Rawls cannot find any data to work from. And a search of the literature shows Philpott to be making more claims than scientific evidence can support at this time. Philpott also promotes his own magnets and may therefore be biased. This is not to say that these claims are false; however, more scientific research confirming or disproving these claims needs to be done.

The only study to date on this issue was published in the September 1990 issue of the *Journal of the National Medical Association*. Scientists took petri dishes full of cancer cells and put them in either the biomagnetic north pole end of a magnetic resonance imaging facility or the biomagnetic south pole end. In three weeks, the petri dishes in the north pole end exhibited a dramatic decrease in cell growth, which is what you want to see with cancer cells. The dishes in the south end exhibited a slight, but detectable, increase in the rate of cell growth. This is the first experiment to address this question, and more work is clearly needed.

To add confusion to the issue, some scientists believe that there is no strong evidence supporting the use of one pole over another. This point of view is especially prevalent in Russia. Japanese manufacturers who uphold this point of view sell magnetic mattress pads that expose the body to both north and south fields, although some experts have warned against this practice.

Dr. Zimmerman is currently studying the difference between unipolar and bipolar magnets in the treatment of lower back pain. The unipolar magnets have flat surfaces and expose the subject to just one field, while bipolar magnets expose the skin to both fields simultaneously. They are designed with alternating spatial patterns of north and south poles, so they may be arranged, for example, as concentric circles, like a target, as alternating squares, analogous to a checkerboard, or as alternating triangles. Both types of magnets have their proponents, and Dr. Zimmerman is seeking to address the issue from a scientific point of view rather than be influenced by manufacturers' advertising.

An argument against the north/south dichotomy is made by Dr. Pawluk, who says that there is no proof that magnet wearers are being exposed to just one polarity. Pawluk questions the existence of a purely north or south field as he talks about the impossibility of the "Bloch wall" (which is the dividing point between north and south poles where there is no magnetic field): "The problem with the Bloch Wall is that in a magnetic field, molecules line up perfectly and produce lines of force that are very strong in one direction. The lines of force bend around and then turn back on themselves. You have one molecule on one side that's lined up in one direction and one molecule on the other side lined up in the opposite direction. When they bend around, they cancel each other out.

"Let's assume the upper part of the magnet is the north pole," Pawluk continues. "Then the bottom part will be the south pole. At the top part, the lines of force are north pole lines. In physics, I'm not sure anyone can make a distinction between a line of force coming out of the upper side or north side of the magnet versus the line of force that's coming from the south side. It's not like cold and hot water. There's no scientific evidence proving that they are different. If you move away from the edge of the magnet by an inch or half an inch, and you measure the area with a magnetometer, you'll find that the field has changed from positive to negative. Say the top surface is positive. If you move one inch to the side, you'll find, when you measure the area with a magnetometer, that the field has changed and become negative. It goes from a north to a south pole. What that means is that at any given time with a permanent magnet you are actually being exposed to both the north and south pole. When you have a very dense magnet, there's obviously a higher concentration of south pole at the surface than there is at the sides. Nevertheless, you're actually being exposed to both fields."

In summation, Dr. Pawluk explains that most scientists now believe that permanent magnets create their effects because of the drop in the field, or what is known as the gradient. The change in polarity may be what is producing the effect in the body. In other words, both north and south poles are entering the body at any given moment, and the entirety of the magnet is what is doing the healing.

How Magnets Are Used

While very little research on magnet therapy has been done in the United States, there has been a lot of work in this field in Russia, Czechoslovakia, and the Western European nations over the past thirty years. This discrepancy parallels an experience I had about fifteen years ago when I approached the FDA to see what information they had concerning glandular implants as a way of rejuvenating body systems. They said there had not been a single study done and that it was quackery. A quick review of the American literature did suggest there was never a study done in the United States. But after going to Vienna, Austria, as well as to Heidelberg, Germany, and interviewing scientists and clinicians working in the field of glandular implants, I was provided with over five hundred studies published in the peer-reviewed literature. Similarly, if you look for research on fixed magnets in the United States, you will find a paucity and think there is a minimum of hard evidence. However, if you were to go to Russia, where magnetism is a well-regarded and highly respected science, you'd find hundreds of studies on fixed and pulsed magnetic therapy. It is rare for an American physicist to read Russian, and hence review their literature. But Dr. William Pawluk has done just that and shares his views in our Clinicians' Reports section, showing that there is more than adequate reason to feel very positive and assured about the nature of this research.

Even if you do not have access to the research, magnets are simple to use. So, why not give them a try? My suggestion would be to use magnets on yourself, as if you were performing a single controlled study. Listen to what your body tells you. If you have had unremitting arthritis pain in your hands and apply a magnet to it, you may find that three days later you no longer have pain for the first time in ten years. Remember, your own experience is valid. This book is an effort to combine practical commonsense usage and good clinical experience. Science will simply have to catch up.

A COMPLEMENTARY THERAPY

Of course nobody is saying that magnets are a be-all and cure-all. They should not be used by themselves for any major disease or medical condition, but rather, they should be looked upon as an adjunctive therapy. My own personal experience is that magnets work best in combination with other healing modalities. Ever since seventh grade, I have been a competitive athlete, winning dozens of USA track and field national championships, regional championships, and over three hundred local races. And I have set numerous American records. Therefore, I know my body well. When I sustained a severe hamstring injury, I used magnets— small, medium, and large, from 500 gauss to 5,000 gauss— wearing them for fifteen minutes at a time and sleeping with them taped to my leg. The magnets hastened my recovery.

A year and a half later, I reinjured the same hamstring. This time, I used magnets in addition to intravenous vitamin C drips, glutathione, calcium, magnesium, quercetin, and other nutrients at very high dosages. The first hamstring injury required almost three months to heal using magnets alone; the reinjury required two weeks to heal. I have seen the same results throughout my career when multiple therapies were used instead of an individual one. Hence, I believe that magnets should be used in combination with other healing modalities, which may include therapeutic touch, acupuncture, acupressure, deep or soft tissue massage, and compresses, to name just some of the approaches available.

WARNINGS

While magnets are generally safe, there are times when they should not be used. Here are some caveats to keep in mind:

Pregnancy. Until research proves otherwise, pregnant women should not wear magnets, particularly over the abdominal area, which would expose the fetus to the magnetic fields. Using magnets on the shoulder, arm, or elbow, however, would not expose the fetus and would be allowable.

Pacemakers. Individuals wearing heart pacemakers or other electronic implanted devices should not use magnets near the apparatus. A magnet should not be suspended over the heart, for instance. Nor should they be worn on the mid-back where the magnetic field affects the heart from the opposite side. It is all right, though, to wear magnetic insoles for sore, tired feed, or a magnetic pad on the elbow, knee, or ankle.

Bleeding Wounds. Magnets lessen the stickiness of platelets, blood components that make a scab after you cut yourself. So, if you use a magnet when you have an active bleeding wound, you may actually increase the amount of bleeding in the wound. It's best, then, to wait until the wound gets sticky or starts to show evidence of healing. Apply magnets at that point. Definitely do not use magnets if you are on antico-agulants or if you have a condition, called polycythemia, that increases the likelihood of bleeding.

Bipolar Magnets for Those with Infections and Cancer. People with cancer or any sort of infection, like candida, fungi, vi-ruses, or bacteria, should avoid exposure to bipolar magnets. As we've mentioned, many believe from their observations and clinical experiences that the south pole accelerates the growth of cancer cells, bacteria, viruses, and fungi. Not all practitioners and manufacturers agree, but until the research proves otherwise, it is prudent to err on the side of caution, and only use products with north-facing magnetic fields.

CONSIDERATIONS WHEN USING FIXED MAGNETS

The effectiveness of magnetic treatment depends large-ly on four factors, according to Dr. John Zimmerman: strength, thickness, number of magnets used, and spacing.

First, magnets vary in strength, and it's important to remember that stronger magnets penetrate more deeply than do weak ones and that the reading at the surface of the magnet is different from the reading at its core. In other words, a magnet that is a 2,000 gauss at its core may only be 200 gauss at its surface. If the problem area is covered by a thick layer of skin—say, at the thigh—the magnet may not be able to penetrate deeply enough to make a real difference. A strong, thick magnet will be needed. To penetrate 4 inches, one needs a 300-gauss magnetic field, and to get that strength, one may need a magnet of about 8,000 or 10,000 gauss at its surface. These are hard to find but can sometimes be purchased through commercial distributors.

Neodymium and ceramic magnets tend to be more powerful than the plastalloy type. In general, the magnets that people should be purchasing are unipolar. They are flat-surface magnets that are magnetized along the direction of the surface. Note that horseshoe and bar magnets are not suitable for therapeutic application, as they are magnetized on both ends or at the ends of the U-shape. Commonly, the magnets used therapeutically are either circular or rectangular. Several can be stacked for increased gauss strength and, therefore, greater effectiveness.

The thicker the magnet, the greater the depth of penetration. The down side to this is that, with increasing thickness, the magnet becomes more uncomfortable to wear. As a compromise, one can wear magnets between $1/4$ and $3/8$ of an inch thick.

Manufacturers often stack a number of magnets closely together in the same direction. The more magnets that a manufacturer includes in its product, the stronger the magnetic field and the greater the depth of penetration.

The final factor in magnet effectiveness has to do with the thickness or spacing of the pad between the magnet and the skin's surface. Usually, this space is pretty small—about an eighth or a quarter of an inch. This spacing makes the magnet more comfortable to wear and also smooths out the bumpiness of the magnetic field.

Dr. Zimmerman explains: "There's a phenomenon called south pole bleed-through. If you have a magnet that's a standard $3/8$ of an inch thick by $7/8$ of an inch wide by $17/8$ inches tall, on one side of the magnet you have the north pole, and on the other side you have the south pole across the surface, $7/8 \times 17/8$ inches. For round figures' sake, we'll call it 1×2. Across this 1×2-inch magnet, one side is north and the other is south. If you take a sensitive magnetometer, and you hold it against the north side, you will read north everywhere along the surface of that magnet until you reach the very edge. At the edge of the magnet, you'll start seeing south pole. That's called south pole bleed-through. Relatively few magnet manufacturers realize this.

"The way to avoid south pole bleed-through has to do with an interaction between this number and the spacing of the magnets and the thickness of the pad between you and the magnet. If you have relatively few magnets spaced far apart—say twelve magnets spaced two inches apart—then you must have a thickness of some substantial amount, say two or three inches, before the magnetic field will become uniform. If you have a dozen magnets in a 3×4 array, in between each individual magnet you'll see the south pole. If you move a distance away from the magnet, say two or three inches, all the measured polarity will be north. There will be no south pole bleed-through. But if the magnets are spaced two inches apart, the thickness of the spacer must be rather substantial, say two, three, or four inches, to avoid south pole bleed-through. That makes the magnets much weaker, and it makes the pad uncomfortably thick. To avoid that, you can place the magnets much closer together. Instead of two inches apart, you can place them half an inch apart. Of course, if you space the magnets half an inch apart, you have to have more magnets. So, instead of having one dozen magnets, you might have three or four dozen. This increases the weight and the cost of the product, but the advantage is that it allows you to use a much thinner pad. In sum, if you space the magnets a certain distance apart, and you have a certain thickness of pad between you and the magnets, you'll get an entirely uniform north pole field."

Zimmerman goes on to say that because of south pole bleed-through, you want the magnet to be larger than the size of the area being treated. So, if you are treating a finger joint for arthritis, a small magnet is needed; if you are treating a large area, like the abdomen, a much larger magnet is called for.

There are more than two dozen magnet manufacturers (see Resources section). Dr. Zimmerman recommends a company in Deer Park, Washington, called Tengam, as an inexpensive source. He also suggests making an agreement with the seller of the magnet to offer a money-back guarantee if substantial relief is not obtained within thirty days. Reputable companies are likely to make and stand behind such an offer.

THERAPEUTIC USES

Magnets have been used therapeutically to relieve pain and discomfort for thousands of years, perhaps even longer than acupuncture, which is over two thousand years old. The first reported therapeutic use of magnets involved the grinding up of a naturally occurring material called magnetite and the application of this in poultice form to uncomfortable areas of the body.

Magnetite makes for a relatively weak magnet by today's standards. But since the earth's naturally occurring magnetic field was far higher in the past (2 to 3 gauss as opposed to $1/2$ gauss today), magnetite crystals may have been stronger at one point in time. Still, this is a weak field by today's standards, as one can easily buy a magnet with an internal gauss strength of 10,000 (1 tesla) or more. Such high exposures do not appear in any way detrimental; at worst, they seem harmless and at best they appear to help a variety of conditions.

Exposure to the earth's magnetic field plays an essential role in our health, a fact clearly demonstrated when the first astronauts returned to earth sick. Their illness was soon attributed to a lack of magnetism in outer space and the problem was subsequently resolved when NASA placed magnets in their space suits and spaceships.

It has since been discovered that in the absence of a magnetic field, the energy level of atoms diminishes. Necessary nutrients become depolarized and unusable. If this condition is permitted to continue, the body can become imbalanced and function improperly. By restoring balance to an organism, biomagnetic therapy can alleviate a number of health conditions. Some of the most common applications of magnets are described below:

GENERAL USES

Relief from Pain and Discomfort. The most common use of magnetic fields is in the treatment of pain, with reports of successful treatment in a wide variety of conditions, including arthritis, rheumatism, fibromyalgia, back pain, headaches, muscle sprains and strains, joint pain, tendonitis, shoulder pain, carpal tunnel syndrome, and torn ligaments.

A noteworthy American double-blind, placebo-controlled study on the effects of static bipolar magnets on the treatment of post-polio pain was recently published in the *Archives of Physical Medicine and Rehabilitation.* The study confirms the effectiveness of magnets in relieving the pain of post-polio syndrome. Another scientific study of similar rigor is being carried out by Dr. Zimmerman, and is looking at the effects of fixed magnets on lower back pain. There is good reason to expect confirmation of what users have been claiming for years—that magnets are an excellent aid to pain relief.

To understand how magnets work to alleviate pain, it may help to look at pain mechanisms in the body. Pain is transmitted along nerve cells as an electric signal. While quiescent, the nerve has a small charge of about -70 mV. A pain signal depolarizes a cell. Magnets appear to raise the depolarization potential of the cell so that the signal is blocked from depolarization, in effect, blocking the pain. Furthermore, the ability of the nerve to send pain is slowed by a magnetic field. These phenomena can aid in the relief of pain throughout the body.

Pain relief may be enhanced when a magnet's negative pole is placed over certain acupuncture meridians. Research and clinical experience show that magnets increase energy (qi) along these points. The combination of therapies works synergistically, so that their combined effects are greater than the sum of their effects would be if they were used separately. In addition, acupuncturists like magnets because they are painless and allow the treatment to continue long after a visit.

Reduction of Inflammation and Improved Circulation. Injured tissue emits a positive charge; placing the negative pole of a magnet over the area appears to restore a natural balance in the following way: The magnet improves circulation, allowing blood vessels to dilate and bring a greater volume of blood flow to the injured area. This helps to bring in natural healers and to remove the toxic by-products of inflammation—bradykinens, prostaglandins, and histamines—all of which contribute to inflammation and pain. Thus, pain and inflammation are diminished and tissue healing is stimulated.

Antimicrobial Effects. Magnetic therapy can help the body ward off such microbial invaders as viruses, bacteria, and fungi. It achieves this, in part, by increasing immune function through the oxygenation of white corpuscles, an important part of the immune system's arsenal.

A magnetic field can also function like an antibiotic by lowering acidity, with the result that microorganisms have a more difficult time surviving. In addition, hormonal production is regulated, altering enzymatic activity and bio-chemical messengers of the immune system. For example, the pineal gland is one large electromagnetic entity. The net effect is to augment the body's natural ability to resist a variety of germs.

Stress Reduction. The recent discovery of magnetite in the cells of the brain helps explain the calming effect of bio-magnetic therapy. A magnetic field applied to the head calms as well as induces a hypnotic sleeping effect on the brain by stimulating the hormone melatonin. Melatonin is known to be antistressful, producing a sedating effect in insomniacs. This finding has led to the manufacture of magnetic pillows and pads designed to provide a sound and restful sleep. A person can then awaken with more energy and fewer aches and pains.

Correction of Central Nervous System Disorders. Dr. William Philpott claims that biomagnetic therapy can help central nervous system disorders. He states that such symptoms as hallucinations, delusions, seizures, and panic can be allevi-ated through biomagnetic therapy without disrupting the patient's mental alertness and orientation. Also, a magnetic field may reduce the need for tranquilizers and antidepres-sants. Magnets have been used as well to stop epileptic sei-zures.

Energy Enhancement. Biomagnetic therapy is known to in-crease general well-being by enhancing energy. The normal polarization of a positively charged nucleus with a negatively charged outer membrane permits a cell to function as a healthy entity. However, as the cell performs its daily functions, it becomes depolarized. Depolarized cells equal a tired person. It is believed that magnetic energy has the ability to penetrate all facets of the human body and reach every cell. That translates to greater energy and vitality throughout the body as a whole. Consequently, supplemental biomagnetic therapy can help revitalize the body.

One normally revitalizes biological energy during sleep. This can be enhanced by sleeping in a magnetic field. Then, anabolic hormones, such as melatonin and DHEA, are made. Melatonin, made by the pineal gland, is a master hormone controlling the entire energy system.

Quicker Healing. The medical community has known for years that pulsed biomagnetic therapy promotes the healing process, particularly of bone fractures. For over forty years, many doctors have used pulsed biomagnetic therapy to treat fractures and have had a high rate of success. Several magnetic instruments have already been FDA-approved and sanctioned for both safety and therapeutic implications.

The success of this therapy is attributed, in part, to its facilitating the migration of calcium ions and osteoblasts to heal broken bones in less than the usual time. In addition, the migration of calcium occurs away from joints to reduce painful arthritic joint inflammation. The end result is the noninvasive promotion of natural healing, without the use of unnatural chemicals and drugs. Adequate magnetic energy also softens or eliminates scar tissue formed during the healing process.

Some doctors put magnets into the dressings over fractures. In fact, one veterinarian I know, who broke his ankle after falling from a horse, reported using this strategy on himself.

Increased Athletic Endurance and Performance. For years, magnetic therapy has been used around the world on race-horses to heal injuries and enhance performance. Doug Hannum, owner of the Equine Therapy Center in Camden, South Carolina, employs magnetic blankets along with other natural healing modalities on animals, and professional riders, such as five-time Olympian Bruce Davidson and world championship rider Dorothy Trapp, ship their steeds to Hannum for therapy.

Stunning successes with animals have prompted professional athletes to use magnets. The Russians may have been the first in recent athletic history to have adapted magnetic therapy to foster greater athletic strength and achievement. Today, many notable American athletes embrace this technology as well. Denver Bronco linebacker Bill Romanowski revitalized his aching body by sleeping on a magnetic mattress pad. Yankee pitcher Irabu plays with dozens of magnets stuck to his body. Top golfer Jim Colbert endorses magnets. And professional football player Steve Atwinter, a seven-time pro bowler, says, "I am not waiting for scientists to bless it. I only know it works." Even high schools are turning to magnetic therapy to improve athletic performance.

Although the effect of increased endurance and performance is known, the cause is not definitively understood. It is felt that magnetic energy warms up the muscles and joints so that performance is increased. At least as important, serious injuries are reduced. In addition, it is known that magnetic energy increases blood flow to the muscles, thereby increasing strength at these work sites.

SPECIFIC USES

In addition to its general benefits, biomagnetic therapy may help a variety of specific conditions. This is not to say that magnets will cure absolutely, irreversibly, and indefinitely. How much good they do varies from person to person and depends upon such factors as the depth of the problem, how long the condition has been in existence, and how strong the magnet is.

Also, when using magnets for chronic long-standing conditions, where the tissues have not been getting adequate blood flow, you may at first get an exacerbation of symptoms. Some people call this a healing crisis. The discomfort usually passes in twenty-four to forty-eight hours. In the meantime, one may wish to take some aspirin, or similar pain-relieving medication to help with the discomfort until the body starts to recover its circulation. One alternative is to decrease the length of time the magnet is worn in the beginning and to gradually increase the time.

When using magnets for healing purposes, the strength should generally be between 1,000 and 5,000 gauss. Most treatments employ static magnets. However, when treating fractures, either static or pulsed electromagnets can be useful. Here are some conditions for which magnets can be helpful.

Aging. Magnets activate life-promoting enzymatic activity which, in turn, encourages normal cell division. This creates a healthier organism and may then slow down the aging process. Several studies on animals show magnetic therapy to increase lifespan. In order to balance the energy of the organs and glands throughout the body, it has been suggested that one apply magnetic fields to the whole body. Sleeping on a magnetic bed is an excellent way to accomplish this. Drinking magnetized water is another good habit to get into. Additionally, injured or weak areas of the body can be strengthened by applying magnets to these specific sites.

Amputations. Many amputees suffer from a phenomenon called phantom pain; i.e., they feel pain in a limb that was removed. Many of these patients have vascular problems. Research shows that in many, magnets can improve the flow of blood in the stump and cause phantom pain to go away.

Appendicitis. A northern or bipolar magnet can be placed over the affected area. In advanced infections, however, you should not hesitate to call a doctor, as this is an emergency situation.

Arthritis. Magnetic therapy may be one of the most effective methods for achieving relief from arthritis, according to a recent study published in the *Journal of Rheumatology* (November 1997, p. 1,200). Placing the north pole of a magnet over an inflamed area on a regular basis may be a key factor in improvement, especially for arthritis in the hands and feet. Magnetic therapy may help reduce bone and tissue degeneration.

Asthma and Bronchitis. Wearing a strong neodymium magnet over the chest to cover the bronchial tubes and at an equal level on the back may help these conditions. In addition, sleeping on a magnetic mattress pad can be beneficial.

It may take several days before breathing returns to normal, and magnets can be worn continuously during that time.

Scientific evidence supports the use of magnets in bronchitis, in both adults and children. In his clinical practice, Dr. William Pawluk reported success after a patient of his, who suffered from chronic bronchitis after having been poisoned by mustard gas, used magnet therapy. The use of this treatment resulted in a greater ease of breathing.

Breast Fissures. Breast fissures are skin wounds that occur in women who are breast-feeding. Placing magnets over the wounded skin can help the fissure heal more quickly.

Burns. Magnets can help speed up the healing of all but the most serious burns. They are good to keep around the kitchen for burns received after touching a hot stove or picking up something that is scalding. Magnets should be placed over the site of injury. For slightly more serious burns, the use of magnets may help reduce the need for analgesics to control pain.

Cancer. Cells depolarize before becoming metastatic, and so one can speculate on how this approach may have been successful in those clinical cases that have responded to magnet therapy. When using magnets for cancer, remember the following rules of thumb: The magnetic pole used must be negative. The field should be larger than the primary lesion and the gauss greater than 25. Success rate increases if both the gauss and duration are increased. A minimal duration of twenty hours per day for no less than three months is required in most cases. The therapeutic effect is, in part, a result of the negative pole producing alkaline hyperoxia (abundance of oxygen). Cancer cells form their energy by making ATP in an acid anaerobic environment, which is termed acid hypoxia.

Russian reports indicate that using magnetic therapy along with chemotherapy increases success in the treatment of brain tumors. Patients given magnetic therapy were less sick than patients who did not receive it, and they recovered more quickly. They also had fewer problems with their adrenal glands, which chemotherapy can sometimes affect.

Since the amount of information available on magnetic therapy with cancer is so limited, and since cancer is such a serious condition, one should never consider magnets as a sole therapy.

Carpal Tunnel Syndrome. Magnets can be applied to the front and back of the wrist to help this hard-to-heal condition. While the symptoms can be controlled with the help of magnets, one should not expect the condition to be automatically cured.

Cervicitis. The Russians have designed magnets for intravaginal use to alleviate chronic cervicitis. They are placed in the vagina, next to the cervix. While this method may be useful for chronic cervicitis, it probably should not be used for acute infections, such as yeast infections.

Circulatory Problems. One can place magnetic strips along the forearm and sleep on a magnetic pad at night.

Depression. When magnets are placed over the head, they can help lift one's mood and promote relaxation.

Dermatitis. As magnets decrease swelling of any kind, they can be placed over any area of inflamed, red, itchy skin with favorable results.

Ear Pain. Magnets can be placed over the painful site. Medical advice should also be sought, though, particularly for children.

Endometriosis. This painful condition causes infection and inflamation inside the pelvis and is characterized by tissue irritation, inflammation, and pain. Women with infertility problems often suffer from this. Benefit can be realized through magnetic therapy, although it might take several months. In one study, good results were seen when 250-gauss magnets were placed over the lower abdomen for six to twelve hours.

Fibromyalgia. One should sleep on a magnetic mattress pad and use a magnetic pillow. Magnets can also be placed over painful areas during the day.

Foot and Leg Problems. Magnetic insoles will increase circulation and help conditions such as numbness, burning, aches, restlessness, and leg cramps. In addition, one should sleep on a magnetic mattress pad.

Head Injuries. Head injuries, even mild ones, can leave people with chronic, debilitating problems, many of which show up years later as headaches, memory disorders, chronic fatigue syndrome, eye problems, irritability, or other symptoms. Magnets placed around the head and neck can correct the electrical imbalance precipitated by the injury.

Heart Disease. A neodymium magnet worn over the heart may assist, along with a lifestyle, diet and stress magnet program, the body in healing itself, and may, in time, allow one to lessen or discontinue medications. Of course, one should always follow a physician's advice.

Some of the effects of magnets on circulatory function are greater blood vessel dilation and increased oxygenation of tissues. Biomagnetic therapy may also improve vascular resistance and decrease the stickiness of blood platelets. People with a peripheral vascular disorder and arteriosclerosis may therefore benefit from magnetic therapy. Biomagnetic therapy may also undo blockages throughout the body, such as in the vessels of the lower extremities, the arteries in the neck, and the blood vessels in the hands and arms. By opening up a blockage in the heart, magnets may help prevent or improve ischemic heart disease, angina, and heart attacks.

Muscle Spasms. One of the major actions of magnets is to decrease spasms in muscles. If you pull a back muscle or you're under a lot of stress, those muscles may tighten up. Placing small round magnets or little block magnets over those areas can make a significant difference.

Dr. Pawluk reports additional relief when acupuncture meridians are stimulated with magnets: "In some patients, myself included, I've placed a magnetic pad over the sacral area because it hits the bladder meridian going up the back. The bladder meridian controls the energy flowing through the muscles, all the way up and down the back, including, to some extent, the shoulders. If you increase the energy flow along the bladder area, it will help a muscle problem or tension up into the shoulders."

Muscle Strains and Sprains and Joint Pain. Dr. Pawluk reports success after applying a magnet over the site of a torn muscle: "While playing with the family dog, I tore a muscle in my calf. It was very painful. I covered the area with a large magnetic pad, one that was probably 8 × 10 inches wide. And I wrapped an Ace bandage around that. I wore that for three days. It made a significant improvement in the pain and discomfort and reduced the bruising around the tissues."

Local applications are appropriate for these types of problems. Wear the magnet for several hours, and then take a break from it. Either wear the magnet all day and take it off during the night or vice versa. The same rule applies to joint pain. A magnet can be taped over the joint for a set period of time. Additional benefit can be derived if magnets are placed over corresponding acupuncture points.

Inexpensive Radio Shack magnets can be very effective when worn over the site of a local strain or sprain.

Neuritis. The Russians performed a study of thirty-nine neuritis patients on medication alone, and an equal number on medicine plus magnetic treatments. Magnets were placed along the spine, even though the neuropathy may have been experienced in the arms. The assumption was that some of the information processing originated in the spine. Therefore, treating the spine would be reflected in improvement in the arms. The experiment found a great degree of improvement in both groups, but particularly in the group receiving medication plus magnetic treatment. Pain was reduced and nerve reflexes improved.

Post-Polio Syndrome. Recently, a study was performed examining the effect of bipolar magnets on post-polio syndrome, a condition characterized by muscle tenderness and pain in patients who have had polio. The condition occurs years after the original damage from the polio virus. Application of magnets to these tender, painful spots was shown to alleviate pain in this double-blind placebo-controlled study, the results of which were published in the November 1997 issue of the *Archives of Physical Medicine and Rehabilitation.*

Rheumatoid Arthritis. Magnets act as an anti-inflammatory, and therefore help some chronic inflammatory conditions, such as rheumatoid arthritis.

Surgery. Some studies have shown that using magnets for twenty-four to forty-eight hours before surgery, over the site where the incision will be made, results in better postoperative recovery. Additionally, wearing magnets over a wound after the sutures have been put in can also speed up healing.

LENGTH OF EXPOSURE

In many studies using magnets, patients experience favorable results with intermittent use as opposed to continual wear. In other research and clinical experience, conditions are alleviated when magnets are worn full time. This raises questions for further research: Should magnets be worn all the time or should they be worn for certain intervals? Should the length of time they are worn vary from condition to condition or person to person?

Dr. Pawluk asserts that research shows that if magnets are worn all the time, the body may adapt to the field and establish a new level of homeostasis. This can be compared, Pawluk explains, to walking into a room that has the scent of flowers. After one is there awhile, the smell becomes imperceptible. The body may, therefore, need a periodic time-out from magnets.

CLINICIANS' REPORTS

Doctors and other clinicians who have been using magnets for years have a lot to tell us about what this treatment modality can accomplish. Here, in their own words, are their reports.

Dr. Michael Tierra

In the last four years, I have been using magnets on thousands of patients and I have found them to be the treatment of choice for inflammation and pain. I have never seen any other therapy work faster to relieve arthritic pain, lower back pain, joint pain, and most other conditions.

The strength of the magnets I use regularly is no less than 3,000 gauss. Normally, I use small magnets, called Acuband magnets. They are applied topically and simply stuck on with a special adhesive strip that a person can leave on for a week or two. They stay over the site of the pain or inflammation even when the person is showering.

The most important thing to learn about using magnets therapeutically is that they have north and south poles. The north pole is basically that side of the magnet which is attracted to the north. (This is the conventional definition of north, contrary to how biomagnetic north and south poles have been defined throughout the text.) For therapeutic purposes, that's called the north-facing magnet. That is the yin side. It promotes circulation, and disperses—and basically relieves—pain and inflammation. In most cases, that's the side that therapists find to be most responsive in the treatment of infectious and inflammatory conditions of all kinds. For chronic conditions, however, where energy is needed at a particular site to relieve underlying stress and pain, the south-attracting side is often necessary.

I think it's important that people understand the differences between north and south because if you use the south-attracting side inappropriately, for instance on tumors or on an organ that's expressing a lot of congestion, it will make the condition worse. If you use the north-facing magnet on someone who has a more chronic condition, it can also make the condition worse.

One of the questions people ask me is, "Do I need to use magnets constantly, or do they actually promote a cure?" Basically, I use magnets to relieve acute symptoms. Along with that, I use herbs, diet, acupuncture, and so forth, to enhance the healing process. It's been my experience personally that when magnets are used for a long enough period of time, which is variable for each person, they do, in fact, have a permanent curing effect on the areas that they're intended to treat.

Let me tell you about how I got started using magnets. A couple of years ago, I had a rather chronic, acute knee problem, for which I tried acupuncture, herbal packs, and many other therapies. I had magnets sitting around in my office, and I wondered about how to use them. Previously, I had applied magnets to patients, with varying results. I think the reason was that I wasn't using them correctly. Anyway, in desperation, I decided to apply the magnets to my own knee. I simply stuck one on my knee over the trigger point. In about two hours, I noticed that the pain was getting a little bit worse. Realizing that magnets have north and south polarities, I took the magnet off and turned it around. When I placed the north-facing magnet over the pain, within two hours the pain was 98 percent gone. My knee was so improved that I was able to take my son to Disneyland. At the time, I was working one of the trade shows in Anaheim, and it was rather embarrassing to be standing in my booth, a cripple, with knee pain. Yet with the magnet I was able to function completely. I was pretty amazed.

Experimenting over the next two weeks, I would turn the magnet around, applying the south pole, and I would find that the pain would worsen. Then when I would turn it to the north, the pain would disappear. It seemed like magic. Usually, I'm a skeptic, but the power of magnets, in my own particular situation, was absolutely astounding.

From that point on I became intrigued. I realized that I was on to something, and I started using magnets with all of my patients. I applied the north-facing side of the magnet on patients with elbow pain and carpal tunnel syndrome. I saw people with chronic neck pain from whiplash recover. I applied magnets topically over an ovarian cyst, and I saw the cyst shrink and dissolve in three or four months at most. I learned that chronic or acute back pain is usually very simple to treat with magnets. The pain usually leaves within one to three weeks. I found magnets incredibly effective for the relief of sciatica. They could also help when there's been disc degeneration. In fact, it's more the exception than the rule when people with joint disorders and pains and lower back pain are not relieved with the use of magnets.

I've also used them for coughs by fixing a north-facing magnet at the pit of the throat. For asthma, magnets are phenomenally effective. Placing a magnet between the seventh cervical and first thoracic discs, and the areas next to it, on a horizontal plane, about an inch out from the spine on either side, has been effective in about 95 percent of all asthma patients I have treated. I've also found magnets to be very effective for gastrointestinal problems and headaches.

One case was really amazing. A woman with colitis came to see me. She had bleeding ulcerative colitis for over a year. I didn't know whether magnets were going to work. But I was on a mission to use them on every single case that came along. I identified a trigger point below her navel and applied six 2-inch north-facing magnets horizontally over the area. These were Acuband magnets with a strength of 6,000 to 9,000 gauss. When she came back a week later, she was almost completely free of pain with no sign of any blood discharge.

I've even used magnets on skin diseases, which was a real test because skin diseases are not usually localized. Being so pervasive, it's hard to find a trigger point, a place where you can place a magnet. However, in most eruptive skin diseases, there is one locale where the condition is more concentrated. It's like the head of the dragon. Applying the north-facing side of a magnet on that place would literally cut the head off, and the surrounding areas of skin would then clear up. This has worked for eczema, psoriasis, and even shingles.

One of the most astounding cases was a person with a brain tumor. His X ray and EKG diagnoses showed that he did indeed have a brain tumor. Based on the work of Dr. Philpott—he has done a great deal of work on the use of magnets with cancer patients—I applied the north-facing side of a very strong neodymium magnet. Since he had to wear the magnet 24 hours a day, I had him wear it in a cap over the area where the X ray showed the brain tumor was located. This went on for about three months. I didn't know whether it was doing him any good or not. He eventually went home to France and had X rays and an MRI of the brain which showed that the tumor had shrunk. It wasn't completely gone, but it had shrunk considerably. I think this is absolutely amazing.

It's important to remember that when treating a tumor the north-facing side of the magnet should be used exclusively, only the strongest magnets should be used, and they should be worn consistently.

I think the core of magnetic therapy is seeing people with problems get immediate relief after being exposed to a low magnetic field. Recently, I was interviewed on the TV show *Inside Edition*. A patient was in my office at the time. She was an airline stewardess who suffered from chronic tendonitis of the elbow, from lifting trays. The woman had no idea as to what I was going to do. While the television crew was setting up in the next room, I placed the north side of the magnet on the elbow—usually I use the north-facing pole first. I specifically looked for the trigger point and placed the magnet over that spot.

I learned something intriguing about magnets. That is, when you put them on, and you move them, you can get an immediate healing response if there's going to be any at all. I've seen magnets alleviate pain in about 85 to 90 percent of cases, and I've used them in hundreds of pain and inflammation cases over the last three or four years. But never before have I been able to establish that people will get a healing response within two or three minutes. I think that is absolutely startling. I put the magnet on, and then I lightly tapped on it about 30 or 40 times. At first, I put it on with the north polarity, which is the one effective for most people; it's the yin or the anti-inflammatory side. But her pain actually got worse. Then I thought, maybe she needs the south polarity because it's chronic. So I turned the magnet over and tapped on that. Within two minutes, she felt better. I had her challenge her elbow. I literally tried to make it hurt, but the pain was completely gone. It was at that point that I called the television crew in to film her in her excitement. The pain that she had for years was literally lifted away within two minutes.

I've been able to demonstrate that many, many times now. When I wrote my book, I didn't know about that particular technique. My subsequent editions will have an appendix that describes this technique as an experiential way to determine whether someone needs a north or south pole. It sounds like magic, and it sounds strange, and believe me, there's nobody more critical about things in the alternative movement than me. But if something works I am not going to deny its authenticity. I can't say why it works, just that it does. When something works, science needs to find out why it works, not whether it works.

Personally, I think we're in the dawn of a magnet revolution. In two years, I believe that magnet therapy is going to be one of the hottest things going in the United States. Here, it's just beginning to surface in most people's awareness. I think where people are beginning to take notice of magnets is with athletes. Athletes generally have a problem of reinjury because they don't stop; they're competitive, and they don't allow themselves to heal properly. By using magnets, they can relieve pain, promote healing, and increase circulation so that they can continue to perform.

Magnet therapy is simple. Every time I give a lecture on it, I tell people that all they need to know is the correct use of the north and south pole. And that can be told in about 10 minutes.

While there isn't a lot of research on magnets, I'm hoping that the National Institutes of Health will designate some of the money that they have for alternative research for it because magnets do incredible work and you don't need to know a whole lot to use them. It's a fact that over 10 million Japanese people sleep on low-gauss magnetic mattresses every night. A few Japanese studies show absolutely no negative effects from the use of magnetic therapy whatsoever. In my own experience, I've used them on just about everything you could imagine, and I have not seen any negative effects.

Doctor "Joe," M.D.

I have been in private practice since 1973. Before that, I spent two years in the Air Force as a physician on active duty after medical school and residency. I graduated from the University of Cincinnati's College of Medicine. I finished my urology residency at Ohio State University in Columbus. Then I went into the service for two years and started a private practice.

I've been involved with magnets for approximately three years. . . . I had a back problem. . . . I could not stand or sit for more than an hour at a time without my back really hurting. This had been going on for 18 years. It was a non-surgical problem, but it was very annoying and sometimes very debilitating. At least once a week, I would have to take Tylenol with codeine in order to sleep at night. I was on nonsteroidal drugs for five years.

I started using some magnetic products. Within three days, most of my pain melted away. I am not taking any pain pills now for my back for over two and a half years. Nor am I taking any anti-inflammatories.

Does my back still hurt? Yes, sometimes. And I just apply the magnets for two hours for a day or two, and things settle down. So magnets really have changed my life.

I started using magnets in my practice for anything from minor aches and discomforts to [more troublesome] problems. Three years ago, I had one fellow in his late 30s . . . He had injured his back in an industrial accident five years before that. He was totally disabled and on worker's comp. He had had two major back surgeries, which had not really done a whole lot. He was on all kinds of pain medications. He could not sleep at night. He was doped up with pain medicines. He had just come back from his neurosurgeon who told him that there was nothing at all that they could do. They were going to send him to a pain clinic to get injections in his back, which he didn't want to have. He was suicidal. He started using magnets, and within a matter of three months, believe it or not, the man went back to work at his old job.

I have many stories. . . . A couple of years ago a woman came into my office. She was in her early 60s, very slim, maybe 5'9" or 5'10". She was all hunched over with a cane, dragging one leg. I asked her what the problem was and she said that back in 1983, she had been diagnosed with fibromyalgia. Another name for it is chronic fatigue syndrome. She told me she had been to several famous clinics and had

seen all types of neurologists, orthopedists, physical therapists. She was on over $200 worth of pain medication a
month. She said she couldn't sleep for more than an hour
and a half without waking up with pain. She would stay in
bed until one in the afternoon because she wasn't getting any
sleep. She had a wheelchair that she was using at home.
Basically, the woman was bedridden.

We gave her a magnetic mattress pad and a pillow. Two
weeks later, she and her husband came back. I asked her
how she was feeling and she told me that she felt better than
she has felt in a long time. I asked her what she meant and
she said that the day before she took half the amount of
medication that she normally takes. She said that the first
night she took the magnetic mattress home she was able to
lay down and sleep for six hours straight. She said the second
night her husband fell asleep on it. Her dog used to follow
her around all the time. Now she wasn't able to get the dog
off the mattress. Another thing she told me was that she
forgot her cane. They have since bought a larger mattress
pad, keeping the smaller one for the couch.

This was almost three years ago. I saw her back this past
summer for an infection. She's up and about and tells me
that her husband won't let her get rid of her cane and her
wheelchair. They're in the basement. She's now on absolutely no medication at all.

Let me tell you a dog story too. One of my [magnet]
distributors down in Dayton had a dog that was 10 or 12
years old and had arthritis really bad. The dog would sleep
with her in bed, and in the morning just crawl out. When
the dog hit the floor he would cry from hurting so bad. She
had just got half of a magnetic mattress pad for her side of
the bed. The first night, the dog would just randomly sleep

on one side or the other. After the second or third night, he started to sleep with her on the mattress pad. About a week or 10 days later, the dog gets up in the morning, jumps down out of bed, and runs away.

I don't know how magnets work. But I'm a very practical and pragmatic person. It really doesn't matter how it works; the only thing that matters is if it does.

Of course, the earth is a giant magnet. It has a north pole and a south pole and a solid core. It rotates around and creates a magnetic field. All living organisms, from day one, have evolved in this magnetic field. I'm told by scientists, and from what I've read, that over a period of the last 4000 years, the earth has lost approximately 90 percent of its electromagnetic field. We live in houses that have wires running through them. We work in buildings that have steel girders in them, that have fluorescent lights, that have televisions, computers, and so forth. All this creates an electronic smog that further diminishes the earth's natural magnetic field. I think the reason we're having so many chronic problems with aches and pains and arthritis and this sort of thing is simply because we aren't getting enough magnetic energy that is basic for life.

When the astronauts first went into space, they came back with what we call space sickness. They thought that was due to the lack of gravity in space. The Russians knew about this a little bit before, and then we found out after doing some elimination, that they were out of the earth's natural magnetic field. The astronauts, even if they were up for a short time, were coming back with all sorts of muscular problems, losing calcium from their bones, and that sort of thing. They thought it was gravity. Then they started to simulate the earth's natural magnetic field by putting magnets in their space suits as well in space capsules. And they eliminated about 90 to 95 percent of all the problems they had.

We need magnetic energy. It's like we have a run-down battery. Then we put the insoles in our shoes, and we sleep on the pads, and so forth. And basically what it does is it recharges us and gives back what we're lacking.

Dr. Ronald Lawrence

My experience with magnets goes back about five years. I was a skeptic and thought as many M.D.'s think. I thought that magnets were quackery. But I decided to try them in double-blind studies with patients. Overall, my results were astounding. Eighty percent of cases were helped. And what were those cases mainly? I found magnets to be very helpful for arthritis, particularly degenerative arthritis, which is the more common wear-and-tear type arthritis. I found them to be excellent for pain problems involving muscle spasms, not as much for acute pain problems as for chronic pain problems, such as chronic sprains that athletes develop. I found them to be excellent for low back problems, tennis elbow, and mild carpal tunnel problems.

About three years ago, I did a study on 22 carpal tunnel patients and found 80 percent effectiveness in the early stages. This led me to believe that magnets may have a preventative effect in this repetitive stress injury to the wrist, which is so common nowadays.

They are extremely effective for pain problems. I'm a specialist in pain and had the first in-patient pain clinic in the United States.

I became interested in the use of magnets because magnets really have no side effects. Of course, I don't recommend them for people with cardiac pacemakers. As a matter of fact, the magnetic resonance imaging (MRI) machine, which is in common use, has a minimal strength of 15,000 gauss. It's been shown that there are no biological side effects from that. So magnets don't really cause side effects. I like that idea of no side effects and an 80 percent effectiveness rate for pain and swelling.

Placement is extremely important. When a joint is affected, magnets should surround the joint. If you're going to use magnets on the knee, I suggest a minimum of four placements around the knee to get the desired effect. The same with the elbow and the wrist . . . [the magnet should put out] a reasonable field strength, which should be somewhere in the neighborhood of 400 to 500 gauss. The main thing to remember is to bind the magnet tightly to skin so that there is a very small air gap. Also, the magnets should surround the area you're trying to affect.

Magnets have been used with great effect over acupuncture points. I have been an acupuncturist for the past 25 years and can tell you that magnets work to enhance health when placed over these points. They're very effective for the lower back, for example, when placed one inch parallel to the spine, on both sides. There's a very important point between the first finger and the thumb called large intestine 4. When you place a neodymium magnet—which is a tiny, powerful magnet—over this point, you'll get changes which alleviate headaches.

I've been in practice for over 45 years, and there are few things that excite me. I've been excited about acupuncture and the whole field of alternative health, of course. But few things have excited me as much as magnets. . . . I started to see the results.

Jim Joseph

Let me begin by explaining how magnets work. First of all, they normalize pH, the acid/alkaline balance, which, in turn, creates an internal environment that is conducive to good health. Sick people, regardless of the disease they have, are almost always in a highly acidic state. Pathogenic activity loves acidity and the hypoxia (low-oxygen) state it creates. The negative pole of a magnet effectively addresses this issue.

Magnets bring in oxygen. They help to optimize oxidative ATP, and this, then, helps in the production of healthy cell growth and replication. At the same time, magnets inhibit fermentation ADP, a substance needed by pathogenic activity for its energy production. So what we're really seeing here in the latter part of the 20th century is pathogenic activity getting a leg up because of low oxygen and lots of acid in the body. And that's where magnets come in very, very effectively.

Magnets also pull aberrant calcium off of cell walls, and we have a lot of free calcium excess from the acidemia. That free calcium excess is related to chronic inflammation and connective tissue breakdown. We see this in arthritis, fibromyalgia, rheumatoid arthritis, lupus, and so forth. And we create oxidative stress with this free radical proliferation.

When our blood passes through a negative magnetic field, we repolarize each cell. That accelerates the cell's electrical spin. We're speeding up electron activity, causing cells to repolarize and break apart so that we don't have platelet aggregation and cell aggregation. Keep in mind that only one cell at a time can slip through a capillary, so we increase capillary activity and circulation, we carry out toxins and bring in nutrients. We're increasing the body's effectiveness and productivity on every level.

Another thing that magnets do very effectively is activate enzyme systems. Our enzymes are under an enormous amount of stress from [our] eating too many dead, denatured foods. These foods are deficient in life-promoting enzymes. Magnets encourage greater enzyme activity, and they promote normal cell division.

Magnetized water is a powerful healing agent. Do this by placing the negative pole of a magnet on one side of the water and the positive pole of a magnet on the other side. In as little as five minutes, you will have bipolar magnetic water. However, I keep my magnets on all the time for a very enhanced magnetic water.

By magnetizing water, you increase oxygen's productivity. Keep in mind that oxygen is paramagnetic. It therefore picks up negative magnetic energy, carries it into our bodies, and distributes it, helping to alkalinize the body.

One of the protocols I suggest for many illnesses is sleeping on a magnetic bed. It's analogous to lying down in the earth's magnetic field and bathing our bodies in that healing energy. At night, we're in a catabolic state, as opposed to an anabolic one during the day. And the body's recharging, if you will, healing, and bringing in oxygen. I also suggest putting 4 × 6 magnets on your headboard. They project about 18 inches, bathing the head, and the pineal gland, which is a magnetic organ. This, in turn, gives rise to melatonin production. We've heard a lot about taking melatonin. That has value. However, we could have a biofeedback mechanism where the body, thinking it has enough melatonin, shuts off melatonin production. By using magnets, we keep the pineal gland actively producing melatonin. So bathing the system in a negatively charged magnetic field all night is wonderful. I generally find that people can get two hours less sleep, and rise more restored and refreshed.

The other thing that I suggest to repolarize the body is to take a 4 × 6 positively-faced magnet, put it under your left foot, and put a negatively-faced magnet under the right foot. In about 15 minutes, you will rebalance the body's polarities.

As you see, magnets help our systems overall, but for specific problems it's important to know how to place magnets locally and how to supplement magnet therapy with other healing modalities. Let's look at several common conditions.

For bronchitis, an inflammation of the lining of the bronchial tubes, I suggest that people put the magnets directly over the bronchi. For a severe inflammation of the bronchial area, it's good to put the magnets on the front and the back. If the area is large you can use plastiform magnets. These come in 12-inch strips. They have 4-inch widths, and they're about an eighth of an inch thick. You can run these from the bronchial area all the way up above the collar bone, across the chest. They can be stacked for extra depth of penetration.

This will bring in oxygen, which will diminish viral and bacterial infection as well as environmental contaminants. It will also quiet down the inflammation. When we have inflammation we have pooling and acid. Acid is a very strong component of this kind of infection. So we're alkalinizing the area. We can place three or four stacked plastiform magnets over the area with an Ace bandage. Or we can be creative, placing them in shirt pockets. That way you don't have to wrap around the body.

Keep in mind that the negative pole should always face the body. But you don't want to have negative magnets over the thymus for an extended period of time because it sometimes can mitigate thymus activity. The thymus is right in the throat area. You don't want to wear these for 24 hours a day on the thymus; you want to give the thymus a chance to rebalance its polarity.

I also want to caution anyone with a pacemaker or any defibrillator not to use magnets, as they can disturb the electrical energy output of those devices. Another caution: Even though there have not been any problems with pregnant women or fetuses, there are no studies in this area. So [perhaps] erring on the side of safety, I would say that pregnant women should not be using magnets.

The protocol for bronchitis would also be effective for colds and flu, particularly where it's affecting the lungs. Magnets here have a very strong antibiotic effect. I would suggest doing this for 45 minutes, once a day, and then sleeping on a magnetic bed pad for 8 to 10 hours.

If you are really sick and don't want to get out of bed, I caution you not to spend more than 8 or 10 hours on a magnetic bed pad. It can be enervating in terms of energy production, and also affect the adrenal glands.

If you have any diarrhea with the flu, it's good to stack four 4×12 plastiforms across the transverse colon. Or you can even sit on the magnets. I have found that to be extremely beneficial for people with severe diarrhea, even long-term cases.

I always suggest magnets as one of several protocols. It's also important to eat a reasonable diet and to take herbs like goldenseal, echinacea, and astragalus. In addition, it's helpful to drink 8 to 10 glasses of negatively charged healing water for its antibiotic effect.

Moving on to bursitis, the first thing to consider is food sensitivities. Wrong foods can produce a lot of acid. They can create free calcium excess, chronic inflammation, and connective tissue breakdown. To help stop that, you can place a magnet right on the area of bursitis—a lot of people have that around the shoulder area. You can use a wrap that will hold six or eight magnets. That will greatly increase penetration into the area. I'll take a 2 × 5 or 4 × 6 and stack it on top of one of those patches and wrap a bandage around that. I find people get almost immediate relief doing that. I find that using a higher gauss of 3900, and stacking another magnet on top of that (up to 5600 gauss), for short periods of time, has a very powerful clearing effect. It clears out the congestion in the area and heals quite dramatically.

Sometimes you'll find bursitis in the elbow or hip. There are elbow wraps and hip wraps that you can use. Be especially careful with the elbow. You want to put the negative field on the elbow. On the other hand you don't want a strong positive field against your body. So you have to keep your arm away from your body. There are also knee wraps and ankle wraps, which I suggest wearing for about 45 minutes once or twice a day.

Bruxism is the grinding of the teeth at night. Usually, there's a calcium/magnesium deficiency related to that. And very often there's an emotional component. If left untreated, bruxism eventually breaks down tooth surfaces. If you want to relax that whole area, you can stack three or four 2 × 5-inch plastiforms at the base of the head. That's in the occipital area. It will relax the whole emotional area. Or you can also place round ceramics at the temporal lobes at the sides of the head.

While we're in that area, why don't we talk about temperomandibular joint (TMJ) problems? What we can do is put a magnet one inch in front of the ear canal, where you have that little indentation. That will relax the TMJ area.

If you have a toothache and you can't get to a dentist right away, you can put a magnet over the painful tooth. Use a neodymium. Its penetration is low, only about 2 inches. But its gauss strength is high, about 12,000. Keep in mind, you must use the negative pole. Placing that over an area of pain in the mouth will help pain to subside rapidly.

The oral cavity is a diagnostic window to the body. Where we have cavities, we have receding gums. I see so many people who have arthritis and pain in their joints, and they all have periodontal disease, every single one of them. It's predictable. What's happening is they have acid in their body and acid in their mouths. Mercury is also acid-producing. Magnets are very effective in turning around the acid in the mouth and at disengaging the calculus from the bones and teeth. Instead of scraping and digging in the teeth, you can repolarize. Calcium is positive. With magnets you can create a negative field that actually pulls the calcium off the area. There are toothbrushes that are magnetized that do that very effectively.

We're a constipated society, and a lot of it has to do with the standard American diet. It's from a lack of fiber, from being highly stressed, and from not paying attention to your body. Very often depression is involved. I see it as the inability to get one's life moving. Diverticulitis and hemorrhoids can also come from that. What you need to do is stack three 4 × 12 plastiform magnets—plastiforms mold to the shape of the body—over the transverse colon. That's across the body, a little below the belly button. That will draw water. Remember, the negative field pulls energy. So it pulls fluids and gases, and draws water into the area, eliminating dehydration. It will soften the stools and ease elimination, definitely helping hemorrhoids as well. This should be done premeal or an hour and a half afterwards. Otherwise, you'll eliminate the peristalsis action of the colon.

If you don't have plastiforms, you can sit on a 4 × 6 ceramic magnet. That will bathe the area in the negative field. These magnets are a half-inch thick with a penetration power of about 18 inches. They will also bring liquid into the area.

In addition, remember to drink sufficient amounts of water. People generally don't drink enough. If you drink distilled water, magnetize your water. . . . Keep in mind with distillation we eliminate minerals, and we need to replace them. Store water in glass jars.

Vitamin C will further help loosen stools. Since there's a direct relationship between low fiber and constipation, drink green juices, putting back some of the fiber and "chewing" the juice.

Diverticular disease is far more common in the west than in so-called underdeveloped countries. For this, you need to put a minimum of three plastiform magnets over the area of pain for at least 25 minutes. Avoid laxatives. They only exacerbate the problem, and make for a lazy colon. The best laxatives are whole, live, natural foods, with an emphasis on greens.

Edema, or fluid retention, is a symptom of other problems, such as heart or liver disease. Paradoxically, you might not be getting enough water as the interior of the cells are giving up fluid in a reverse osmosis way and flooding the extracellular area with fluids. I would suggest using negative magnetic energy to pull that fluid up from the area. If it's in a lower extremity, put the magnetic energy above the site of the edema, and toward the kidneys. It will pull that fluid up and away from the site of injury. In severe cases, you can put a 4 × 6-inch magnet on each kidney. You can also use wraps. Always keep in mind that the magnet should be placed above the site of the edema.

For hyperthyroidism, an overactive thyroid, you can wrap the thyroid. This is the site of the Adam's apple in men, and the same area of the neck in women. You can put one round disk magnet on each side of that throat area to bathe it in negative energy. That will slow down the thyroid's thyroxin production. I would suggest using an 850-gauss ceramic magnet for 25 to 40 minutes.

Our livers are constantly under assault. They have to process enormous amounts of toxins, the result of too much animal fat, chemical toxins, food sensitivities, parasites, liver flukes, and alcoholism. The liver's a very large organ, so a 4 × 6 inch negatively-poled magnet would be excellent here. It would help to alkalinize and oxygenate the area. Parasites are not going to enjoy the oxidation or alkalinity that the magnet will produce. If you're not getting results, you can stack two 4 × 6 magnets to get a strength of about 5600 gauss.

The liver is located on the right side, just under the rib cage. It runs all the way across, almost to the belly button. If you have extreme problems with the liver, you can put a magnet directly behind it so you're bathing the liver in negative magnetic energy. You can slip the magnet into a pocket of an old shirt and wrap the shirt around you.

Along with magnets, there are several important measures you should take. Drink green juices. Go back to a plant-based diet. Avoid alcohol, sugar, and processed foods. And use the herb milk thistle. Along with magnet therapy, this is an effective program for detoxifying the liver.

In lung diseases, such as emphysema and cancer, we need to place magnets right over the lung area. With cancer, you must cover the entire tumor with a negative field. The magnet should be worn as close to 24 hours a day as possible in order to exhaust the energy of the tumor. All pathogenic activity, including cancer pathology, makes its way through ATP, through what is known as a substrate process or fermentation. You therefore want to create an environment which will make it impossible for pathogenic activity to continue. Cancer cells do not like oxygen, so we want to superoxygenate the area to make it inhospitable for any kind of disease to exist. Do this by stacking 4 × 6 magnets over the area. In addition, employ every healing technique possible. Work on your attitude, use guided visualization, eat a plant-based diet, and so forth. I find attitude to be the number one thing here. When I work with people, I find that once they have the proper attitude, they take the necessary action, and they become excited about life.

One of the nice things about magnets is that you can put them in your medicine cabinet. They are always available, and they don't ever wear out.

Dr. Goldflies, orthopedic surgeon

I'm a board-certified orthopedic surgeon. I've been in private practice in Chicago since 1981. A special interest of mine is endurance athletes. I have been treating runners, cyclists, and triathletes for years. My interest in sports medicine and in taking care of these athletes led me to magnet therapy. Actually, I heard about it at a sports medicine meeting several years ago. The athletes who were using them first were racehorses. We started using them on our human athletes and found similar results. I've been using them for five years now with significant success.

Years ago, when people were getting MRI scans, some would come back afterwards and tell us that their pain would go away for several days and then slowly come back. In orthopedics, we were using bone stimulators which pulsed magnetic fields through bone and would allow for healing. There were several theories as to why this worked. It appears from some of the newer basic science research that a pulsed magnetic field increases microscopic circulation to the tissue. That affects healing. It improves the oxygen to irritated muscle and tendon, thereby stopping inflammation. Also, by opening up the microscopic circulation it enhances blood supply to an irritated or damaged area. So our basic application for magnetic therapy in practice now involves several things. First, for acute problems, for either soft tissue sprains or fractures, especially around the foot or ankle, we find that placing a magnet over the affected area, either applied locally with taping or even incorporating it in a cast, appears to decrease pain and swelling. It appears that people get helped much more quickly with magnets.

We then started applying them to more chronic soft-tissue problems, like tendonitis, arthritis, bursitis. We would palpate or push, finding the area of maximum tenderness, place the magnet over that area, and within five days we'd know whether or not we had a significant effect. We have found that people with arthritis do well when magnets are used as an adjunct treatment.

One of the more difficult problems I treat is tibular stress syndrome or stress fractures in my runners. Even with the use of braces and casting, some still remain symptomatic. By placing a magnet over the more sensitive area, most of them, within a month, heal up and become asymptomatic.

Several of our patients with fibromyalgia or chronic fatigue find that the magnetic mattress pad improves their ability to rest and get a better night's sleep. It alleviates muscular soreness when they wake. On a short-term basis, we find that it's effective. We warn people, though, that every two weeks or so they need to get off the pad for a few days.

One of my best successes was with a nurse who came in with an ankle sprain. She had the usual swelling and black-and-blue changes. When I mentioned that she should use a magnet she looked at me and laughed. She came back two days later and said, "I took some magnets off of my refrigerator. I stacked them and put them on my ankle. It was much better. Sell me some magnets."

Another story was with a 54-year-old male runner with tibular stress syndrome from running that would not resolve. Within a month of magnetic therapy he improved. Another runner in his 60s had pain on the inner aspect of his knee at the shinbone. It was symmetrical. I actually used him as a guinea pig. I gave him a grid magnet for one leg and a unipolar magnet for the other. He came back a month later, and I asked him which magnet worked better. He said that they both worked the same. The pain was gone and he was running again.

We find that pulsed magnetic fields are the most effective. There was a development of a patented technique for putting a grid, north and south, on one surface of a flexible magnet. Thereby, you get both effects. As the magnet moves on the skin relative to the deep soft tissue you end up with a pulsed magnetic field. For healing, you either use the north side of a unipolar magnet or the grid type.

So we look at magnets as a physical therapy modality. We use locally applied permanent magnets and also have a pulsed magnetic field machine in the office. It's much easier for us to use magnetic therapy now because of the media. Information and articles are now available on professional athletes using magnetic therapy. Also, the magnets are much more available now than before.

Magnets are a hot topic among athletes. A lot of professional golfers swear by magnetic devices. There was also an article in *Sports Illustrated* recently on a Japanese pitcher who now pitches in this country with magnets on his forearm. He's convinced that that's the reason he does so well.

William Pawluk, M.D.

I am a board-certified family physician in practice for about 15 years. Trained in clinical epidemiology, I decided, in 1987, to get some extra training in various alternative medicine modalities. I decided on hypnosis, acupuncture, homeopathy, and nutritional counseling. While studying in UCLA's program, I became aware of other cultures using magnetics, in addition to, or instead of, needles, for stimulating acupuncture points. I began incorporating them into my practice in 1992. I know that a lot of people are phobic about needles, so I became involved with magnetics, and lo and behold, I found that people were benefiting.

In order to better understand what I was doing, I researched magnetics and found a ton of scientific literature. A lot of that research was done in the 70s and 80s, when science was looking at ways to do less invasive diagnostic work. With the information I found, it became evident that the body is an electromagnetic apparatus. Since the body is electromagnetic, the question becomes, how can you influence the body's electromagnetic field? Recently, several books have been published giving basic information on how magnetic fields influence biological systems. The best one is *The Handbook on the Biologic Effects of Electromagnetic Fields*, by Polk and Postow (CRC Press).

My interest is electromagnetics, which is more powerful than static magnetics. Electromagnetics is being used all over the world, but it is not available in this country because of the FDA. People wanting to bring these devices into this country are going to have to go through FDA approvals and clinical trials. So we're talking five to ten years before there are usable electromagnetic devices on the market. In the meantime, fridge magnets can be used to give some relief. For example, a small fridge magnet placed on a tennis elbow spot will give relief to a substantial number of people.

One of my first trials was on myself, where I used some very powerful magnets on my face for a periodontal bone recession issue. I actually overstimulated my acupuncture meridians and could actually feel the stomach meridian on fire. It woke me up in the middle of the night. I took the magnets away. I put them back on and the same thing happened. The interesting thing too was that before I actually got to that part of my course, where I knew what I was feeling, I subsequently realized that I had overstimulated the stomach meridian. That, to me, was a significant validation that magnetic fields stimulate acupuncture points.

From there I got different kinds of magnets and tried them on myself for bruises and sprains and sore shoulders. They worked. One of my first patients was a woman who had two discs in her low back for which she was going through training and refusing to have surgery. She was also taking medication. She had used a magnetic pad on her back, which provided her with some, but not complete, relief, so she started using a magnetic mattress pad. I loaned her one and she wouldn't give it back to me because it was working so well for her. Eventually, she was able to stop the back pad and just use the mattress pad. Every time she came off of the mattress pad the pain came back. It usually took a few days for the pain to go away and a few days for the pain to come back. She continues to get relief as long as she continues to use the magnets. We've learned that magnets won't necessarily take care of a physical problem that has pathology. It may resolve symptoms around it and improve tissue healing, but magnets won't raise Lazarus.

Another dramatic experience involves a nurse who had fractured her ankle. She had to have some hardware put into her ankle because of the degree of the fracture and the strain of the ligaments. She wasn't able to square dance or do any lengthy walking in the mall or any lengthy walking with her husband. I gave her magnetic shoe inserts and she was able to accomplish all of those things while wearing them. Whenever she stopped wearing them the pain would come back. The degree of injury she had had produced enough scarring of the tissues that she was never going to be completely free of pain, but the magnetics made a big difference for her.

I recently finished writing a chapter on magnetic therapy which was accepted for publication in a textbook on alternative and complementary medicine. That will end up in the libraries and probably in the curricula of medical schools. The book will contain formal, scientifically based information so that as the medical community begins to look at alternative medicine they have a reasonable basis for understanding how these things work.

I also collaborated on a book which outlines the results of 340 controlled studies of magnets on animals and humans. The research in East European countries is extensive—they have been using magnetics for 25 to 30 years—and shows significant benefits. Eastern European countries understand this modality very well, particularly the Czech Republic, where their equivalent of the NIH has a whole division dealing with magnetics. Magnetics there is considered a standard medical modality; everybody uses it.

[There is a lot of magnetics research in Russia.] They don't have as good a system for cataloguing information as we do in this country, but it is available. One of the studies involving electromagnetics was very impressive. It had to do with cutting out a patch of skin on the backs of rats and applying magnetic therapy on one group. The rats were sacrificed and the skins of the tissues evaluated under an electron microscope. Various chemical studies were done. They looked at the healing activity on underlying tissues. The rats who were given magnetic therapy, for half an hour to an hour twice a day, healed in half the time. In other words, the healing process doubled.

I have found that using magnets locally and over the corresponding acupuncture point enhances the effect significantly. Some of the Russian research we've recently gotten our hands on says that they're using magnets over the spine at the appropriate spinal level. If the problem happens to be in the lung, and you use it over the corresponding spinal segment, you'll get improvement in the lung. If you use it over the neck for problems in the arms, because the nerves to the arms come through the neck, you will also get some relief in the arms.

The most common applications for magnets are for pain. Sometimes it's reduced dramatically; sometimes it goes away. And often that happens in half an hour to an hour. I've had many patients who have been able to resume dancing activities, like square dancing, because of the magnets. And when people stop using the magnets the pain comes back.

I have also treated myself for irritable bowel syndrome. When life gets stressful I will occasionally get cramps and some diarrhea. To help myself, I will use alternating static magnetic fields. I will sleep on a magnetic pad. When I do that the cramps go away and the diarrhea stops. I've used that many times now and have duplicated to my own satisfaction that it works. I don't take an Immodium at night anymore. I just roll over on a magnetic pad.

Magnets can help a variety of conditions. A friend of mine had a migraine headache. I put a powerful magnet over the acupuncture point on his hands. By the time we were done with dinner the headache was gone. I have a number of patients using tiny magnets on appropriate acupuncture points for helping tendonitis, carpal tunnel, and plantar fasciitis. A pediatrician friend of mine uses magnets with attention deficit disorder and finds that they can help. I've used magnets for back spasms and shoulder tightness. And I've used them on my spider bites. If you leave these bites alone, they'll usually last for about two weeks. They'll get angry, big, tender, and irritating. I've put magnets on them and within half an hour to an hour they're gone.

Dr. Buryl Payne

I got involved with magnets when I heard a lecture by Dr. Ralph Sierra, a chiropractor and electrical engineer from Puerto Rico. That was back in 1977. He invited me to come to Puerto Rico to study with him, which I did several times. Then I began to make instruments that produced magnetic fields.

Some time after that, two chiropractors in Kentucky, Drs. Richard and Mary Brewingmyer, flew up to see me. They were very excited about my instruments, and they taught me a method for measuring every organ and gland in the body to determine whether it was overactive, underactive, or functioning normally. This method is written about in two of my books: *The Body Magnetic,* and *Advanced Magnetic Therapy.* I have a third book that will soon be out, called *Getting Started in Magnetic Therapy.*

I have developed five models of instruments. They vary from pocket size to one that will produce a field all around the bed. One would use my instrument for about 15 minutes, a couple of times a day, for maybe 10 days to three weeks, depending upon the condition.

About 80 percent of common ailments are helped by magnetic fields. Let's look at chronic fatigue. The classical approach in magnetic therapy is to put the person on a magnetic bed and hope that will help. But the real sophisticated approach is to use the technique I have mentioned. You can test every organ and gland in the body and then treat appropriately. I have found that everyone I've tested with chronic fatigue will have every gland and organ out. They'll be out in a flip-flop manner. That is the top may be too active. The next will be underactive. They go back and forth down the body. I treated one woman magnetically for just a week, and she completely recovered. A year later, I spoke with her over the phone. She had had no relapse at all.

Low back pain may be helped as well. There are many causes of low back pain, however, and magnets do not help all of them. For instance, a knee being off can throw the hips off and that can throw the back off. It's important for a person to check the liver and kidneys to see if they are off, as well as the hip and the knee alignment. Probably the feet should be checked too. If those are all right, then magnetic treatments will often help back pain. If they're not okay, you might need to get a chiropractic adjustment first.

I have used magnets for my knee that hurts now and then for 10 years. As an experiment, I put the north pole on for a week. It got slightly worse. I put the south pole on and in two treatments it was okay. One year later I had a slight twinge again and I treated it. So I'm always using them. I have them around my bed. And I have designed a magnetic power pad that I treat water with. I put a gallon jug on it and then I drink the water. As an experiment, I put plants on the pads and watched them grow. Wheat sprouts treated with the south pole tasted sweeter. So I do what I can to make little measurements like that. And I generally find that the south pole has a more positive effect.

My next step is using magnetic fields to see if we can reset the biological clock. I want to see if a full-body magnetic treatment can change that.

Tom Nellessen

I attribute my staying healthy to magnets. I'm a smoker, which not a lot of natural healing people are. I've never been to a doctor other than in 1959 when I went into the army and had to get a physical. So I don't know how healthy I really am, but I do know that I feel good. I'll be 58 this year.

I wear a supermagnet, which is a small neodymium magnet worn around my neck in an Indian medicine bag type of pouch. Normally I wear it all the time during the day. At night, I sleep on three magnets that I put between my mattress and box spring. You can do that for a hundred dollars, whereas if you go out to buy one they can run from $400 up to $5000, depending upon who you buy them from.

I work with Native Americans, who accept magnets better than any other population. That's because it's very natural. Like everything else the magnets [involve] the four elements of life. They're made with earth, heated with fire, mixed with water, and cooled with air. Native Americans are open to anything that's unobtrusive, especially when they see how it works.

I use magnets on my daughter all the time. She had asthma when she was born. Fourteen years ago, we were afraid to use magnets on her because we didn't know how bad she was and what it would do for asthma. But she's fine now. Other than the first year of her life, she's never had any medicine for asthma. I put a supermagnet around her neck, which affected her heart and lungs. And I had her sleeping on magnets.

Magnets will help the body to balance itself. If you are too acidic and you wear a magnet, your body will become more alkaline, the way it's supposed to be. With arthritis, I've seen the calcium deposits totally disappear. I've seen Native Americans who were supposed to go in for bypass surgery. They would wear magnets for a week, and when they were checked again their veins and arteries were starting to open up again. The doctors would let them wait awhile and pretty soon they wouldn't have to go in because it would dissolve the calcium, plaque, and cholesterol in the veins, just like your magnetic water treaters work on pipes.

Mildred Schafer, naturopath

I had a sleeping problem when I was introduced to the Nikken mattress. That solved that problem. I think their concentric magnet—that's a balanced field—is good and relieves a lot of pain.

After my heart attack, I started learning more about magnets. I read several books on magnets. I used a 1500-gauss magnet over my heart, using a balanced field. Plus I used all kinds of supplements. Now, at 79, I still work very hard. I don't use magnets on everything, but they do relieve pain.

As a naturopath, I have been using magnets in my practice. I don't always use magnets, but often I do. If somebody says they have carpal tunnel [problems], I show them how to use the magnets. I use magnets to help people resolve their sleep disorders, along with a lot of other treatments like herbal relaxants and melatonin. Magnets seem to reduce arthritic pain, too.

Dr. David Drake, dentist

About 30 years ago, I belonged to a scientific group in Jacksonville, Florida. We had Dr. Albert Roy Davis give a talk. He and another gentleman, Walter Rolls, were involved in magnetic therapy. They had been giving magnetic therapy to patients for years for all sorts of different diseases. That struck my interest.

Then about two or three years ago, a patient of mine said,

"Two months ago, I couldn't walk in here. I was supposed to have two knees replaced, and I was walking with a walker. My sister said to try some magnets. And now I'm walking." This patient's sister had sent her some magnets to put on her knees. She did so, and within a couple of months she was walking well. She went to her orthopedic surgeon who then told her that she no longer needed to have her knees replaced.

At that point, I went down to Greencoast Spring, Florida, to talk with Dr. Rolls. Dr. Davis had passed away, and Dr. Rolls was carrying on the research on magnets.

I then started using magnets, personally and professionally, and lo and behold, the results were outstanding. I had a severe knee injury and needed to do some mountain climbing. But I couldn't even walk up a hill. I put magnets on my knees, and, by gosh, within a couple of weeks I had no pain. Within a month I could kick field goals. I walked up the mountains. Then I helped patients with dental pain. It even relieved temperomandibular joint pain in one patient.

I became one of the charter members of the North American Academy of Magnetic Therapy. There are about 50 physicians, including three or four of us dentists, some chiropractors, some Ph.D.'s, and some scientists.

I'm convinced that magnets are an outstanding, noninvasive approach to healing. Mainstream medicine probably doesn't want to acknowledge it because it often eliminates the need for patients to return. In fact, chiropractors tell me that they give their patients one treatment and some magnet therapy, and they never see them again.

"Dr. Benjamin," orthopedic surgeon

I'm an orthopedic surgeon, now 60 years old. And I inherited bad vessels from my father. He had every vascular procedure known to man two and three times. My peripheral circulation got so bad I could barely climb a flight of stairs. I had an angiogram done back in March of 1993. It showed an 85 to 90 percent blockage of a major artery above my right knee. This caused me to have such bad cramps that I could barely walk. They did an angioplasty and I was better.

Two years later, it was getting so bad again I could barely climb a flight of stairs. I would go to the gym and do toe-ups. But I could only do 25 without getting a severe cramp in my calf. On the golf course, I could not walk from the cart out to hit the ball, and back to my cart without calf pain. Therefore, I had my membership up for sale.

A nurse friend of mine told me to put magnetic insoles into my shoes. I told her she had to be kidding. I didn't see how they could help. I asked her the price; they were $70. Although that sounds like a lot, she explained that an angiogram was going to cost me $1000. And if they were to do an angioplasty it would be another thousand. If they were to screw up the artery and do a bypass, it would cost me a month off for pain and suffering. I'm a complete coward, and so I said, "Bring the damn things by and I'll try them."

I put them in my shoes without any confidence that they'd do anything for me at all. Within two to three days, however, I walked up two flights of stairs without calf pain. I went to the gym and did my toe-ups. I did 50. Before, it was 25 and I had to stop because of the cramps in my calf. I called the golf course and asked them not to sell my membership.

I have worn the magnetic insoles every day since then, and you would have to fight me to get them out of my shoes.

One day I forgot to put them in my golf shoes, and I started to get worn out. My legs started to hurt when I walked. I did not realize what I had done until I got back in to change my shoes.

I wear them every day. I did 60 toe-ups at the gym last week before I had to stop because of calf pain.

How do they work? I don't know. I don't care. It doesn't make any difference to me if it's a placebo effect. I haven't had to have surgery.

I then went to a wellness meeting and another orthopedic surgeon was making a presentation. He was the brother of the nurse who got me to put these things in my shoes. I listened to his presentation. After he told me how he uses them on his patients I signed up and became a distributor. I bought all these magnetic devices. They were sitting in my office. I had no clue as to how to use them. They just sat there collecting dust.

One day, a little over two years ago, a patient came to see me who had no joint cartilage left. I had him scheduled for a total knee replacement. He kept delaying surgery and wanting more and more Vicodin every day. He was taking six to eight in a day. I figured this guy was going to Betty Ford after he fixed his knee to get off the stuff.

My X-ray tech/surgery assistant said to me, "Why don't you put some magnets on his knee?" And I thought, Why not? It can't hurt him. So, I took two little round, silver-dollar-size magnets and taped them on the medial collateral side of his knee. I forgot about it.

I went to one of our magnet meetings three weeks later and saw my patient. I said, "What are you doing here?" He said he wanted to know how these things worked. I asked him about what happened, and he said that since I put those magnets on his knee, he was having no pain. He had no need for Vicodin. He also mentioned that he had called my office to cancel his knee replacement surgery.

Since then, I've put these devices on 300 to 350 people. I have them write me a check for the value of the product. I do not cash the check for 30 days. If they're not happy with the product they can bring it back and I'll give the check back to them. Eighty percent of the people keep the magnets. They want them. And I cash the check. Twenty percent bring them back. And the 20 percent of the magnets that come back look brand-new. In other words, I don't think they got used.

Do these things work? The answer, in my opinion, is yes. It's hell yes. It's not accepted by the FDA; it never will be. The reason they will never be FDA approved is because the people who make [pain relievers] will damn well see to it that this is never FDA approved. That would put them out of business.

Fred Turner, physical therapist

I use magnets a lot for treating back pain. I have a magnetic wand that I use occasionally on people for that purpose. I use magnets for arthritic thumb conditions, for people who have fallen and who have some bruising on their hips, and for shoulder injuries.

Patients don't seem to mind trying magnets because it's pretty well publicized now. First, we try it in the office, and then we let them take it home. If they get results we let them use it for a long period of time at home.

I used magnets on a back problem of mine. I would place a large magnetic pad in a lumbosacral brace and wear it for a day or two. Then everything would be fine.

A most interesting story has to do with an arthritic thumb that I have. As a therapist, it makes it difficult to write and work with patients. As a result, I put a magnet on the meta-carpal joint of the thumb, and it relieves the pain almost immediately.

I have an 82-year-old mother who fell down the stairs. I put it on her hip, and in two days' time she was able to walk a mile.

Dr. James P. Elmes, orthopedic surgeon

I have been using magnets for many years for various problems. Originally, I used them to help speed up the slow healing of bones. And I used post-magnetic fields to overlay casts in fractures that were not healing.

More recently, they've developed static magnets for vari-ous pain problems. These fit on the skin with a strap, and are placed over the painful area. Magnetic pads are left in place until the pain goes away, which can take anywhere from several days to a couple of weeks.

Magnets are used for many types of problems, such as musculoskeletal types of pain in the head and neck area in cases of cervical arthritis. I use them for bursitis and ten-donitis in the shoulder and for various headache problems. People have had success with tennis elbow, various forms of arthritis around the thumb and wrist, carpal tunnel prob-lems, and lower back problems. Many golfers use magnetic wraps for back problems. They're also used for bursitis prob-lems around the hips and knees, and tendonitis around the ankle. Magnetic inserts that fit in the shoe are helpful for heel spur problems.

One patient of mine, a schoolteacher with an arthritic

finger, puts a tiny magnetic pad over the finger with a piece of tape. Within 20 minutes, she starts feeling relief from pain. She will wear the magnet for several days until the pain completely goes away. Then she will take it off and use it again when the pain reoccurs.

We use little magnetic pads over tender spots until the pain fades. One man had both shoulders equally bad. He put the magnetic pad on his right shoulder and kept it in place for about two weeks. He didn't have one for the left shoulder. In two weeks, the pain was relieved on the right side, and he could raise his right arm over his head. But the left shoulder, which had not been treated, did not change. He could not raise his hand above shoulder level without severe pain.

I belong to a group called North American Academy of Magnetic Therapy. They do a lot of work with magnets for the treatment of pain problems. We had a meeting in Los Angeles in the past week. One presentation was with a magnetic mattress for fibromyalgia, which is a problem of multiple pain flurries, mainly in women. They were showing promising results with this difficult-to-treat condition.

I wouldn't say magnets are a cure-all. Some people get complete relief; sometimes there are gradations of relief. Quite often people will get to where they have tolerable discomfort, where they can still do activities that they enjoy doing. They'll feel the pain, but it's something they can better tolerate. They'll be able to do more activities of daily living.

Magnet therapy can cut down on the need for medication. We try to minimize anti-inflammatory pills as well as pain pills and muscle relaxants. Magnets help to minimize medicine, and, also, to minimize injections of local anesthetics.

The main advantage of magnets is that they're a simple modality to use. They help most people, but even when they don't help, they don't do any harm.

Russell Hognowski, massage therapist
I am a massage therapist who incorporates magnetic healing into my practice in Virginia Beach, Virginia, and Hawaii. My biggest success was with a client who had been in a serious car accident 25 years before coming to me. The misfortune resulted in a severed right radial nerve, which, in turn, caused all loss of feeling in his right arm.

After sleeping on a magnetic mattress pad for one month, feeling returned to his arm. That's the best result that I have seen.

In Japan, one out of six households uses magnets. I would love to see the same ratio used in the United States because magnets are a safe and effective way to treat pain and injury.

PATIENTS' EXPERIENCES WITH BIOMAGNETIC THERAPY

In the following section, people who have benefited from the therapeutic use of magnets describe their experiences.

Barbara, on relief from sciatica, headaches, and toothaches

I had sciatic problems, off and on, for a long time; it was serious for two years. After I got it pretty well cured, I noticed over the years that when I got stressed it would come back and ache. I began to wear magnets and found they would take away the pain. In fact, I found them to take pain out of almost anything.

An abscessed tooth that is really bad requires pain pills and a trip to the dentist. But if you use magnets when you first find out about it, they will draw the pain out. If I have a bad leg or ankle, I put [a magnet] on.

God designed magnets. The entire universe has magnets in it. I live without pain because of them. Never do I fail to have one in my purse. It gets rid of a headache so quickly that you can't believe it. It pulls the pain out. That's all there is to it.

Tom, on grandson's healing after dog attack

Approximately a year and a half ago, my grandson was attacked by a pit bull. He had a laceration which took 250 stitches on the side of his face to close. Magnetic therapy was prescribed for that. The healing was so good—the plastic surgeon naturally took credit for it—I've never seen anything heal like that in my life.

Roland, on magnetic mattress pad and elbow injury

My experience with magnets is that I have a magnetic mattress pad. As a video editor, I am exposed to electromagnetic radiation through the equipment I use pretty much all day long. The pad allows me to rebalance my energy at night. I feel that I get a more restful sleep with a magnetic mattress pad.

Also, weeks back, I slipped and fell in my bathtub and really banged my elbow quite severely. I was in a lot of pain. So I rested it on a black magnet, which I had on my desk, for two or three days while I was working. The pain left and it healed quickly. Today, my elbow is totally fine.

Peter, on recovery after a tooth extraction

My only experience with magnets was when I had a tooth extracted about six months ago. I used the magnet in the night while I slept, a single magnet of 3900 gauss. Two weeks later, I went back to the dentist, and he said, "Gee, it looks like it's healing very well. How long was that taken out? About six weeks ago?" I said, "No, two weeks ago." He said it was amazing and I suggested he try magnets.

Lee, on relief of muscular tension and becoming a more alert driver

I've used a few different magnetic products over the past two years. And I've used them extensively with incredible results. The first one is I've been sleeping on a magnetic mattress for most of the past three years. And I replaced an earlier one with a heavier-duty one. My girlfriend, who is a certified shiatsu massage therapist, noticed that prior to my using a magnetic bed it was very hard for her to work on me because the muscles were so tense. It was difficult for her to get through the muscles to the pressure points. After using the magnetic bed steadily, it made my muscles much more accessible so that she could get to the pressure points and be much more effective.

I have a magnetic pad in my car. I often get sleepy driving, especially if it's for more than an hour or two. Since I got a magnetic pad for my car, I find that I'm much more clear when I'm driving, so I've become a much safer driver.

Vicki, on computer protection and pain relief after car accident

I sit in front of a computer all day. I have found that sitting on a magnetic pad makes me feel more energized and less tired at the end of the day without any aches and pains from sitting in one position all day.

I've also found that magnets helped me after a car accident. I put a high-gauss magnet under my pillow all night. When I would awake in the morning I would have less pain than if I didn't sleep with the magnet. It helps relieve the pain of the whiplash throughout the day as well.

I've found magnets useful for many types of pain, including toothaches, back pain, and menstrual cramps, and I've found that with my animals or with myself or my family, just applying a north-pole magnet to the area helps the pain lessen or go away.

Cindy, on asthma, Bell's palsy, and spinal problems

I'm a psychologist who has studied nutrition and other methods of healing over the years, mostly due to my problems. When I was a teenager I had asthma and started looking into herbs. I've sort of been my own guinea pig, so to speak.

About 10 years ago, I started to look into some books on magnetic therapy. Amazingly, the magnets broke up the asthmatic condition that I had. A magnetic pillow helped to increase the mobility in my neck, and it decreased the pain in my lower back. I wear a magnetic strip in my shoes that keeps my lower back balanced. Everything relates to the spine. If I injure myself by doing something I shouldn't do, like lifting something heavy, I use magnets, and they seem to help right away. And they seem to do a very good job. Using magnets helps me to feel better. I can stand longer and my feet don't hurt. I have greater mobility and an easier time exercising.

My husband has Bell's palsy, a terrible, terrible thing. He has bad eyes, but he lost more sight in the eye on the side of his face that was affected. Somewhere along the way, we decided to try magnets. He used a magnetic pillow, and in four days he regained that sight back. He felt that he got the full range of motion back in his neck from using the pillow.

I believe that a lot of us are suffering from a magnetic deficiency syndrome because the earth is losing its magnetic force. We're surrounded by electromagnetic radiation, and we're not grounded on the ground. We're up on the eleventh floor, and we're on cement, instead of being on the ground and receiving the benefits of the magnetic resonance of the earth. I believe that magnetic products help to compensate for a lot that is happening to our bodies. I believe magnets balance out our bodies with what we're being exposed to daily. I think that magnets are still a little bit odd to some people. But I believe that within five years or so they will become commonplace and get the respect they deserve.

Monica, on back problems, fractures, and migraine headaches

I was first introduced to magnetic therapy in a seminar that my husband and I went to in Phoenix. He had a back problem and had been to all kinds of doctors. He had an MRI done and could not sit down at all for eight months. He would have to kneel in a plane or in a car. Back surgery was scheduled for the following week.

One of his friends called him up and asked him to come to his office. A man was going to be coming in with magnets. At the time, my husband was willing to try anything to avoid the back surgery. So we went down there and the man strapped a magnet onto my husband's back. He sat down in his chair normally as the man explained how the magnets worked. My husband is very skeptical and started to argue with the man. Then the man asked, "How does your back feel now?" and my husband said, "Wonderful."

So, he leaves the office with the magnet on his back, continuing to wear it for one or two months. His back completely healed. He doesn't need surgery. So that's our first experience with magnets.

After that, we started to buy magnets. My son had a broken arm and we put a magnet inside the cast. His arm healed probably three weeks quicker than it normally would have.

I use magnets for treating migraine headaches. I put them on the front of my head, and I lay on one. Within an hour and a half my headache's gone. Usually it would take two days to get rid of them.

I also have a hip problem. My hip gets sore from running. This happens about once a year, and I just put the magnet on my hip while I run, and for a week, and then the problem's gone. Now, whenever my kids fall down, they want a magnet on their arm or leg or whatever hurts.

I recommend magnets to people all the time. I used to live in a neighborhood with mostly elderly people. My next-door neighbor broke her ankle doing something. She used a magnet for that. And her doctor was amazed at how quickly she healed.

Magnets are incredible. They're a great way to heal without using medicine.

Ben, on recovery from periodontal disease

I used to see the dental hygienist four times a year for my gum disease. The problem was getting progressively worse, and about 10 years ago I had periodontal surgery. For the past three years, I have been drinking from a magnetic cup. Now my dentist tells me that my mouth is clean; I hardly have any plaque. When I brush my teeth there's no blood from the gums.

Michael, on healing after stitches

Through the years, I have found magnetic therapy to work well in a variety of situations. Here are two examples:

After requiring six or seven stitches for a slash to my forehead, I used a neodymium magnet to speed up healing and reduce scarring. My forehead healed quickly and the site of the stitches is not noticeable.

I find that using a magnetic pad across my legs makes a significant difference in reducing sore muscles after overexertion.

Susan, on thyroid problems, allergies, and dental problems

. . . I started wearing a magnet over my heart. I made absolutely no changes in my diet. Nor did I change my routine with supplements. I wanted to see exactly what the magnet was doing. And I saw some remarkable changes. I saw that my thyroid was functioning better, so I started to wean myself off of my thyroid medication. I came off all of my allergy medication, which I used to take on a 24-hour basis. I would not be without it just in case I should be exposed to a cat or a dog. I have gotten rid of my allergies and I am thrilled. I got rid of my spider veins. That was just kind of a "by the way, look at what disappeared" thing—I was not looking to get rid of them. I noticed an improvement in my circulation, and my immune system seemed to function a whole lot better. I had more energy and I was able to deal with the cold weather better.

Within two weeks of wearing it, I looked in the mirror and said, "What is this? I'm getting new hair in my forehead? And it's brown, not gray? What is this?" My girlfriend says,

"Don't you think you're a little old for long hair?" "No, I like it. And it's growing great." And my nails grow great. They're my pride and joy.

I used to have major dental problems. My parents used to bring me to an orthodontist for low-income people, and I got the guy who should have flunked out. I saw him for 7 years. When he finally took the braces off, all the metal and cement in my mouth caused more damage than good. I ran into a lot of dental problems from that point on to the point where when I was having colds, and flus, and infections, I would go through a lot of tooth abscesses.

One time I was having a root canal done in the front of my mouth. I had an appointment three days later and I started developing an abscess on the side of my mouth. I [said], "Oh, no, I can't go through another root canal at this point. I'm barely getting through this one." At that point I was still experimenting with magnets. I took no pain killers. I took no antibiotics. I did a super peroxide rinse, stuck a magnet on it, and went to bed. I got up the next morning with no swelling, no pain. I never called the dentist for help. Three days later, I went in for my regular appointment and said, "Doctor, you're never going to believe this but . . ." Poke, poke, prod, never hit the ceiling, perfectly relaxed. Poke, poke, prod, nothing. "Let's check it with an X ray just to make sure." He came back scratching his head, poking and prodding again. I was still perfectly relaxed. Then he showed me the X rays and said, "I don't understand this. According to this, you did have an abscess. You don't have one now." He couldn't understand it then, but now when I see him he says to me, "Hey, I just saw another article on magnets." Or, "I saw something on TV." He's getting into it.

Richard, on problems with back and knees and grandfather's diabetes and arthritis

I have played contact sports all my life and have problems with my back and knees. I've had great response with magnets [placed over these areas].

My diabetic grandfather has not felt his feet in years. He used to break his toes and cut his toes, not knowing it until it was too late. But by using [magnetic] insoles, he's been able to get healing back in his feet. It took about a month and a half.

My other grandfather has arthritic fingers. They were broken playing baseball when he was in college. His last two fingers haven't moved in years. He started to use neodymium magnets on his joints, and was able to get mobility back into his fingers. . . .

I've been involved in the magnetotherapy industry for over three years. And I've had many personal experiences. Even people who said to me up front, "I'm going to buy this to prove you wrong because I know it's not going to work" have become big supporters of the products through their own experiences.

I think it's a very exciting time because people are learning that a pill or a shot isn't necessarily the only answer. I've had personal experiences where I've seen such joy in people's eyes from being able to get rid of pain without having to go through great expense and labor.

George, on tennis elbow

In March of '96, I bought a new house. It was on three quarters of an acre that was really overgrown. So I spent two days out there with one of these gas-powered weed eaters.

In doing so, I developed a condition that for lack of a better term they call tennis elbow. It was from having my elbow locked in one position and holding up the weight of the machine. I couldn't even lift a cup of coffee with my right arm, and I'm right-handed.

I went through traditional types of therapies. I went to an orthopedist who told me I needed physical therapy. I went through six weeks of physical therapy, including electrical stim and ice and exercise. It was not any better whatsoever. I went back to my doctor, and he sent me through another six weeks of physical therapy, again with the same results.

At that point, I switched to a different doctor who said, well, about the only thing we can do is try one of these arm exercises. If that doesn't work we'll have to use surgery. You'll lose the use of that arm, more or less, for probably six months. They have to go in and do a bunch of stuff and it takes time to build it back up.

At that time, I was looking into magnetic therapy. I talked to a gentlemen from Norso Magnetics over on the east coast. He said he thought he could do something, and he made an elbow brace that was loaded with magnets. I wore that for about three weeks, but to no avail. So I called him, and he said the problem may be that I was wearing a static magnet which could not get enough magnetic power down deep enough into my arm to solve the problem.

He sent me a Magnessage. It looks like a flashlight, and it has batteries in it. It has a small vibrator motor. And then in the cone, where the light would normally come out, he has three or four magnets. When you turn it on it vibrates. And if you put it up to a gauss meter, you measure the gauss on it with it turned off, and it barely registers. And when you turn it on the light goes bright red on the gauss meter.

I started using that three times a day, just massaging it over the area.

Within two weeks, I had no pain, except when I exerted myself. I had total use of my right arm with no pain whatsoever. If I go out and do too much over the weekend, and it's sore when I get done, then I get the Magnessage out. I'll use it for 15 minutes twice a day for a day or two. All the pain goes away, and I'm fine again. To go from the [only] alternative being surgery to this was truly amazing.

My wife is a competitive horse rider who had persistent problems with her lower back. She sleeps on a magnetic mattress pad, and it helps her tremendously. She usually leaves a magnet on for three weeks out of the month.

Joanne, on back and foot problems

I was having trouble walking. My dentist asked me if I had heard of magnetic therapy, and I said no. He said a man was coming in to talk to him about it on Friday. Would I like to listen? I did. Then I tried it. I found that I was able to walk much more easily with magnetic insoles in my shoes. I wore them all the time. Then I got a big magnet for my back. Whenever I had pain I would put it there, and the pain would go away.

Artie, on low back pain

I used to get up in the morning with low back pain. I thought it was the bed, so I got a new mattress. But that didn't work. I still had lower back pain.

I'm not one for seeing doctors because I believe the body can heal itself when given the chance. My daughter suggested I try a magnetic cushion, and I did. I leave it in the car and use it for long-distance driving. I drove all the way to Florida with it. It's fantastic. I use it at home whenever I'm sitting at my desk for a long period.

A new world has opened up to me. I've just about eliminated all my back pain. Every once in a while I get a little pain, but it's nothing to talk of.

Valerie, on back problems, foot pain, and leg spasms

After I wrote an article in *Success* magazine on multilevel marketing, someone called to say that I should write about a company that he was associated with, a magnet company. I had never heard of magnets used therapeutically, and it sounded fascinating. I asked if there was some way that I could try the magnets first to determine whether or not I wanted to write anything. As it turned out, I ordered some magnets for myself and also for some friends who had various problems. I asked them to try [magnet therapy] to see what they thought about it. Everyone got marvelous results.

I had a leg with bad circulation. It would spasm in the middle of the night. With magnets, the spasms stopped altogether. Some of the symptoms my friends overcame included extreme back problems. Using magnets on the back relieved a lot of the discomfort. Some of them had foot pains. With magnetic insoles, they felt great again. They also seemed to have more energy. Someone else had a very sore shoulder from playing tennis. The magnets also helped relieve those problems.

Rick, on strained ligament

About seven years ago, I was at a conference at Johns Hopkins in Baltimore. The conference was given by a Bill

Pollack, assistant professor of rheumatology. He spoke about a new application, biomagnetics, that they were investigating for soft connective tissue pain. At the time, I had a strained medial collateral ligament in my left knee from skiing. I applied the pad and was shocked. Do you say it's cured? Do you say it's healed? I have no idea. I just know that I have no pain.

After that I started looking into magnets. To make a long story short, I ended up doing some clinical studies for Magnet Systems, a California company that owns a patent on linear alternating bipolar fields. We studied 144 patients with pressure-sensitive pain, back in 1994 and 1995. The criterion for getting into the study was to identify a painful site. If moderate pressure applied with the finger to the site caused pain, the person was allowed in the study. Subjects had carpal tunnel and other kinds of repetitive motion injuries. They had osteoarthritis and rheumatoid arthritis.

The study took five days. During that time, patients filled out a pain assessment form. On a scale from 0 to 10 they rated their pain prior to magnetic application, then 24 hours afterward, and every 24 hours after that for five days. They also wrote any comments down. We compared various magnets, the so-called unipolar, either north or south pole, or the bipolar fields, in various patterns. We tried to come up with a fairly clear picture of which magnetic field, if any, had any influence on the pain. We also used placebos. We were pretty surprised. All of the magnets, as a matter of fact, had a degree of effectiveness, although we do feel that the alternating fields were quicker in relieving the pressure-sensitive type of pain that we were dealing with. We came to a conclusion that magnets had about a 78 percent effectiveness on pain on day one.

I still use magnets today. In fact, I just took some off of my back. And I'm using one right now that I find to be very effective. There's a certain type of magnet that we had developed. We wanted something that was dynamic field rather than static field, meaning something that was dynamic and able to move around rather than stay in one permanent position. It's a very powerful magnet with an awful lot of gauss in it, probably 1500 to 2000 gauss. The magnet rolls around on the inside of a little capsule. Whenever you move, it creates a dynamic field because it's fluxing the magnetic field. I find that that works faster for me. I have discomfort where most people hold their tension, in my upper back above my right scapula. I have a knot that forms there. About twice a week I put them on. I put two of them on, as a matter of fact, very close together. That seems to work most effectively for me.

Mark, on headaches

About 11 years ago, I was in an automobile accident and was diagnosed as having acute cervical strain. The discomfort in my shoulders and neck region brought on massive headaches that sometimes would last for days at a time. Sometimes it would get so bad that I wouldn't be able to function.

A veterinarian I knew used industrial magnets in his vet practice and he successfully treated one of our farm animals. He let me use it for my headache one time, and it seemed to help. I was rather concerned, however, about the safety of the product. There seemed to be a lot you had to know about how to use it.

Then he introduced me to products that were designed

for human use. They were made in a way that was easy and safe for people to use. I had tremendous results.

Steve, on wife's sprained ankle

We used magnets on my wife's sprained ankle. Before we applied the magnets, she wasn't able to walk without the help of crutches. After 10 or 15 minutes, she got up and walked across the floor like nothing ever happened. She couldn't believe it; she was amazed. My wife's an RN, and she had been skeptical about the magnets initially. But ever since that time, she's been supportive.

Many people object to magnets, saying that people who think they work are experiencing a placebo effect. But magnets have been used on animals. Are animals experiencing a placebo effect? A dog, a cat, or a horse knows absolutely nothing about that.

Ben, on father's stroke

My father suffered a severe stroke in October of '94 and had been under full medical supervision with little or no effect. He was deteriorating to the extent that he couldn't even do a jigsaw puzzle. In January of '95 we heard of magnets. So we tried a magnetic seat, and we noticed a slight improvement in my father's energy level.

After two or three days of this, we then decided to put my father on a magnetic mattress pad. We had to carry him onto it. My mother recounts that this was the first time he actually slept through the night.

The following morning, he woke up and he was completely alert. His mind was apparently back to normal from a condition where he could hardly communicate. He completely flipped back to his old self.

But by 3:00 he had deteriorated again. At that point, we put him back onto the magnetic seat, and his energy level once again rose. A couple of hours later he was back to his old self. I always remember him counting his Roman numerals, which was quite a thing.

We continued to have him sleep on the mattress pad at night and use the magnetic seat during the day. He's basically recovered completely from a very severe stroke.

Betty, on multiple sclerosis

I'm an RN who graduated from the State University of Iowa in 1961. I worked for four years, mainly as a psychiatric nurse at VA hospitals. I did some medicine and surgery also, and worked for the last four years for a pediatrician/allergist in Ontario, Oregon.

I have had MS for 30 years. I had numb spots in the middle of my back and inside my great toes. I was terribly fatigued. I went to my doctor after my fifth child was born, and he said that he couldn't find anything wrong with me. With five little kids you're bound to be fatigued. I went on and had five more children, and got even more fatigued. I was actually relieved to find that I had MS and that I did not have a terminal brain tumor or that I wasn't just lazy or crazy.

The best thing that magnetic products have done for me is give me back my energy. I don't wake up exhausted any longer. I wake up after three, four, or five hours of sleep, six at the most. And I have energy. I get out of bed; and my legs don't cramp; my back doesn't hurt; my neck isn't stiff, and I love what I have seen this do for other people. So it's helped me tremendously physically and emotionally.

I've seen the products give others more energy too. A lot of people with my same condition call me from across the country. If they stick it out long enough, it gives them more energy. Sometimes they say, "I feel like my energy is drained." And I believe that's a detoxifying period.

I've gotten more feeling. I even skied two winters ago. My feet didn't get cold, and I didn't get stiff.

Jane, on tired feet

Magnetic products got my attention because six years of being on my feet in the restaurant business left me with knees that ached at night, and tightened up halfway through the day. The first day I put the magnetic insoles in it was not that way. I had the mobility I needed. I didn't wake up at night trying to find a more comfortable position.

Joyce, on chronic disc problem

My husband made our first magnetic pad himself. We really had no idea what it would do. It's a different type of field than what you get from most magnetic pads. With most pads you get reversing fields. What you could say about ours is it's a pure unidirectional negative polarity pad that makes a restored environmental magnetic field. It works with your body because you can sleep on an environmental amount of magnetism forever with benefit.

I had had a chronic bulging disc problem for over 12 years. When I would get out of bed, I wouldn't be able to stand up straight. I would have to slide my whole body out of bed. I would never move my back without consciously thinking about how I was moving it so that I wouldn't cause any pain or increased injury. That would take me about an hour in the morning. Then it would kind of settle down and allow me to function normally for the day.

After sleeping on the pad for three months, I realized I was getting out of bed easier and functioning better with less difficulty during that first hour in the morning. By six months, the whole problem was completely gone. It changed my whole quality of life. I could lift my grandkids. I could do all these different things. And it has stayed gone now for over eight years. . . .

I continue to sleep on the mattress pad. In fact, we have made significantly stronger mattress pads since then. That was the weakest one, and it still helped. A stronger magnetic field just means that your recovery happens faster. The body runs on energy. When you give it more energy, it can do a better job for you, and faster.

Bernice, on fractures

I was in Mexico when I tripped on a rock while walking down a really rough road and broke my wrist. At the time, I didn't know that I had actually broken it. But I was in terrible pain, so I tried some natural remedies, like arnica, and I used a magnet.

When I got back to the States and discovered that my wrist was broken, it was put in a cast. I used the magnet all the time to heal it. The doctor said I would have to keep the cast on for six weeks and I told him that I didn't think so. When I came back in two weeks he said I was doing remarkably well. By the end of the third week, he was able to take the cast off. But he never was really interested when I told him I was using a magnet. That didn't concern him.

Three years later, I had another accident. I fell in my aunt's nursing home and hurt my hip badly. The doctors insisted on surgery. I wanted to leave and go home, but the doctor said he was not taking responsibility. To make a long story short, I ended up having hip surgery. I began using a magnet immediately, and I told the doctor about it. He said that he approved of it, and that he even put magnets in casts when people requested it. That surprised me. I let him put a magnet in my cast, and I healed remarkably well.

John, on chronic neck injury

I had a chronic neck injury. I had surgery on a herniated disc in my neck about 10 years ago. The doctors did a discectomy where they put a piece of my hip in, and I had the fusion. They cut bone spurs out of my spinal cord. Basically, I had residual effects from that: osteoarthritis, scar tissue, and more herniations. I had chronic pain.

I saw an advertisement for magnets on TV and sent away for them. I put it on one night, and the next morning I felt really good. Magnets help right away if you wear them constantly. They seem to take away a lot of the pain. Since I began wearing them, I haven't had to take any Advil or aspirin to relieve pain. It feels like it relieves all the swelling. But you have to have them on for that effect to take place. I wear them indefinitely. They have a Velcro adhesive to them. I've tried wearing a turtleneck and attaching them to that.

It's a problem keeping magnets on when I'm at work because I wear a collar and tie. That's about the only time I really can't wear them. And at night I try to put them on with surgical tape. . . . They really have helped. The effect is amazing.

91

Helen, on rotary cuff problem in right arm

I've had trouble for about six years off and on. I tried physical therapy, and it seemed to help for a while, but then the pain would come back again. It got to where I couldn't even use my arm to comb my hair.

The magnetic product I bought helped almost immediately. I felt the effect the next day and the day after. I can now use my right arm, which I depend on for many, many things.

Jody, on immobile arm

I couldn't move my arm. I went to the doctor and was introduced to the magnets. I put them on my shoulder. The magnets seemed to help right away. It wasn't too long after I got the patch that I noticed I could move my arms. Now, a month later, I can move my arms freely.

I was also having trouble with my feet where I could hardly walk. For that my doctor gave me magnetic insoles for my shoes, and they're helping my feet.

Linda, on arthritis

I had a fusion on my left thumb because I had bad degenerative arthritis in my joints, which left me unable to use that hand. After the joint was fused, I found out that I heal very poorly. The joint calcified, so my doctor told me to wear a magnet over the area to help with the pain and the healing. So that's what I did. It seems that whenever I take the magnet off and forget to put it back on is when I have pain in that joint. When I put it back on, the pain seems to diminish.

I don't think this is in my head because my problem was

proven. I had no cartilage left in that joint. When I wear the magnet constantly, I have more mobility in that thumb, so it seems to have really helped.

Deborah, on cartilage tear, meniscus tear, and bone damage

I had knee damage, and the surgeon cleaned everything out. Once he did that, I was immobilized for four months. Then I was sent to physical therapy. After I started going to physical therapy, whenever I had soreness in the area where the bone repair was done, I would put a magnet on it. That seemed to help with the pain I was having there.

Any time my knee gets sore now I put the magnets on it. It helps it very quickly. Within a half hour I notice a difference.

Laverne, on arthritic knees

I'm 75 years old, and I have bad knees from arthritis. My knees get to aching so bad.

I would apply magnets to my knees and they would feel better. Now I don't have any pain.

I also have arthritis in my little finger. Once in a while it gets sore. So I took the magnet and put it on there just for the heck of it. I was really shocked because the pain was gone. It might have been an hour or so later that I said, "You know, I realize I don't have any pain in my knuckle now."

My sister-in-law too has arthritis bad in her hands. She has the longer magnets that she's been ordering through a catalog. She wears them all the time because she says that when she takes them off she has the pain. They really are wonderful.

Tom, on hip fracture and knee problems

I had a hip replacement [recently] and a knee replacement about six years ago. I've been using magnetic products for about a year now. When I have any problems, like soreness, I tape a magnet to that spot. About an hour later, I seem to get pain relief. I've been using magnetic pads practically every day, putting them on different parts of my hip and knee. They seem to give me quite a bit of relief. I'd say that magnets have helped me quite a bit in overcoming my discomfort.

Millie, on pain

I have arthritis, and I was full of pain. I could not turn in my bed and I could not sleep. My doctor gave me magnets, and the pain diminished. I wear magnets all the time, even when I take a shower.

My foot hurt to where I could hardly walk. My doctor gave me another magnet, a bigger one. I can't do without them.

Richard, on bursitis

I had a job-related problem. As a pipe fitter, I used large wrenches and carried a lot of heavy pipes. I ended up with bursitis in both shoulders. I couldn't seem to get any relief even though I had gone to several doctors. I had received ultrasound treatments, injections, and all types of medications. Medicines didn't do anything at all, except for the pain-killers.

My daughter was going to Dr. Elmes, who put a 4 × 4 magnet on her wrist. Because they were so cumbersome she didn't care to use it. So I borrowed it from her and used it on my right shoulder. In a week or so I had full extension. When I showed Dr. Elmes he was quite excited about it.

I purchased another one for my other shoulder. It's slowly getting better.

I wear magnets continuously. I wear them in bed and while I'm awake. I even shower with them. I just change the tape on them periodically.

I still have some pain in the arm, but the arm is quite mobile. It's surprising. I used to have my wife help me put my shirt and jacket on because I couldn't raise my arm to get it through the opening. Now I can do it by myself.

Magnet therapy is not a gimmick. I can guarantee that. I was a little apprehensive about it at the beginning. But it did help, and it's still helping.

Ingrid, on heel spur

Several years ago, a physician told me I had a very inflamed and swollen right heel spur. I had been exercising at a gym, but had to stop going due to the intense pain. The doctor suggested a cortisone injection, which was extremely painful. After several visits, suggestions of another injection, and a very expensive pair of inserts, I stopped going altogether.

I went to the owner of the gym, who suggested another podiatrist. I took her suggestion and was again told that my foot was inflamed. She said that I needed to be off my foot for at least 20 minutes, three times a day. This ailment was exceptionally debilitating. I am the mother of four children, and I was unable to do so many things that I had always taken for granted. I was actually crippled with pain and restricted in my ability to just walk.

We had gone on vacation and stopped in North Carolina to visit our friends. As I explained the problem I was having, our friends brought us to Jim Sauder [of Norso Biomagnetics; see Resources section] to try some of the magnets he had patented. I wore them night and day. In two weeks time, I started to feel some results. As I continued wearing them, I realized that the pain was diminishing.

I went back to my doctor, and he was absolutely amazed to see that the swelling had disappeared altogether. He then asked me what I had been doing. I explained that all I had done was wear magnets. I had stopped all other prescribed procedures.

I wore the magnets daily for about 3 years, and I removed them from my sneakers approximately nine months ago. My right foot has been absolutely pain free. I have been walking and running almost two miles a day for the past two years.

Ellen, on pain

I was in such excruciating pain from my knuckles and wrists up to my shoulders. My doctor had me take nine Ibuprofens per day, plus I bought all kinds of ointments which, of course, had no effect at all. I could not use my arms to push back the covers in the morning and had to use my feet. It took ages before I could put my arms into my bathrobe.

I am involved with horses and have known for quite some time of the results of using magnetic pads on horses with injuries. I was so desperate I was even thinking of trying one of those for myself when just by chance I happened to hear an advertisement [for magnetic products].

After a few days with a magnetic mattress pad I stopped

taking the Ibuprofen and no longer used any more oint-ments. My doctor was amazed at the difference. When he first saw me I was hardly able to move my arms and hands and my knuckles were very swollen. When I went in after using my pad I was able to swing my arms and bend my fingers, not to mention the swelling had gone away. The pad had done so much for me that I was able to stop taking the Ibuprofen after about three days.

Carolyn, on knee injury and asthma

In January 1995, I suffered an extensive injury to my knee. I was unable to receive any pain relief from medication and therapy prescribed by the orthopedic doctors. Since using the [magnetic] knee wrap, my pain is completely gone.

I also developed asthma in August 1995. I started using the Pneumo Thoracic Shield and have had very little trouble since. I only have to use it when my asthma is really bad during weather changes.

Elaine, on broken bones

In January, I broke my foot while walking. I had been taking prednisone for 11 years and it had apparently thinned my bones. I was in a cast six weeks. During that time, I placed Magnepods on the cast near the break. When the cast was removed, the bones were healed where the Mag-nepods had been placed, but were not healed in the area where magnets were not used.

About a month later, I fell and broke my wrist in two places. I placed a 2 × 3 magnet on one side of the cast and a 2 × 2 on the other side. After four weeks, the cast was removed and the X rays revealed that the wrist was completely healed.

I showed the orthopedist my magnets and explained how I used them. He said he didn't dismiss [claims of] the effectiveness of magnets because he uses pulsating magnetic therapy to speed healing on broken bones.

Sally, on migraine headaches

I have experienced migraine headaches periodically for many years. Recently, I was driving my car to work when a bright glare from a mirror on a truck I was following blinded me for a second. Soon I was aware of the usual premigraine headache visual signs, including a blind spot in the middle of my field of vision. Thankfully, I did not have much further to drive as I could feel the headache coming on. I worked for 10 minutes or so until the pain began to increase to the nausea stage.

I decided to try the Magnessage to at least relieve some of the tightness in the muscles of my neck and head. After about 15 minutes of use the pain began to recede, and within 20 to 25 minutes the pain was gone. For those of us who suffer from migraine headaches, this really is close to a miracle. I will certainly keep the Magnessage close at hand to try to alleviate future migraine headaches.

What the Future Holds

In the twenty-first century, medicine will change from a field dominated by chemistry and surgery to one that promotes the body's own healing ability, and biomagnetic therapy will surely play a big part in this shift. At present, while magnetism's ability to alleviate a variety of conditions is well documented, we do not completely understand how this happens. So more basic research is needed. We need, too, to provide greater knowledge about how to manipulate magnets for the best effects. As we increase both our scientific and clinical understanding, skeptics in the medical community will be won over to this vitally important healing modality.

A burgeoning field of inquiry involves methods of slowing the aging process. Antiaging research to date has focused on medicinal herbs, hormones, and nutrients that enhance health but do not necessarily lengthen the genetically determined life span. A popular belief has been that each cell has a figurative biological clock that predetermines senescence and maximum life span. For years, scientists have tried to identify the exact nature of this clock, and recently, they seem to have done so. It seems that each time a normal cell divides it loses small portions of the ends of its chromosomes, which are regions called telomeres. When telomeres are shortened to a certain critical length, the cell can no longer divide. This results in the cell growing old and eventually dying.

Part of this divisional activity requires bonding of proteins to each other through a process known as hydrogen bonding. It is known that hydrogen bonds are influenced by magnetic fields, and there is a possibility that magnetic fields can be used to affect hydrogen bonding in a way that will reset the biological clock.

Another factor in aging is a decrease in the production of the hormone DHEA. It is known that magnetic energy can influence hormone production from the pineal gland. It will be interesting to determine if this therapy can influence the production of DHEA, with a resultant slowing of the aging process.

Peer-Reviewed Scientific Studies

Following are descriptions of recent studies, published in peer-reviewed scientific journals, on the impact of treatment with magnetic fields on a variety of conditions.

Alzheimer's Disease

R. Sandyk, "Alzheimer's Disease: Improvement of Visual Memory and Visuoconstructive Performance by Treatment with Picotesla Range Magnetic Fields," *International Journal of Neurosci,* 76(3–4), June 1994, p. 185–225.

This article reports on two Alzheimer's patients who experienced significant improvement in visual memory and drawing performance following the external application of electromagnetic fields ranging from 5 to 8 Hz. Improvements were also seen in other cognitive functions, including spatial orientation, mood, short-term memory, and social interactions.

R. Sandyk, et al., "Age-related Disruption of Circadian Rhythms: Possible Relationship to Memory Impairment and Implications for Therapy with Magnetic Fields," *International Journal of Neurosci*, 59(4), August 1991, pp. 259–62.

Noting that the disorganization of circadian rhythm (the daily biological clock) may be causally related to memory deterioration in old age and possibly to Alzheimer's disease, this article argues that the use of magnetic fields could lead to memory improvement among the elderly by means of re-synchronization, or resetting, of the circadian rhythms.

AMYOTROPHIC LATERAL SCLEROSIS (LOU GEHRIG'S DISEASE)

A. Bellosi & R. Berget, "Pulsed Magnetic Fields: A Glimmer of Hope for Patients Suffering from Amyotrophic Lateral Sclerosis," Second World Congress for Electricity and Magnetism in Biology and Medicine, 8–13 June 1997, Bologna, Italy.

This article reports on three patients with amyotrophic lateral sclerosis who experienced beneficial effects following treatment consisting of three sessions per week of pulsed magnetic fields administered via a Magnobiopulse apparatus. Patients received upwards of 75 total sessions prior to achieving maximum recovery.

ANKLE SPRAIN

A.A. Pilla & L. Kloth, "Effect of Pulsed Radio Frequency Therapy on Edema in Ankle Sprains: A Multisite Double-Blind Clinical Study," Second World Congress for Electricity and Magnetism in Biology and Medicine, 8–13 June 1997, Bologna, Italy, p. 300.

Results of this double-blind, placebo-controlled study indicated that treatment with two 30-minute sessions of non-invasive pulsed radiofrequency therapy is effective in significantly decreasing the time required for edema reduction in patients suffering from lateral ankle sprains.

ARTHRITIS

Y. Mizushima, et al., "Effects of Magnetic Field on Inflammation," *Experientia*, 31(12), December 15, 1975, pp. 1411–12.

This study found that 3 hours of exposure to a 50-Hz magnetic field significantly inhibited experimentally induced inflammation and suppressed arthritis in rats.

J.C. Reynolds, "The Use of Implantable Direct Current Stimulation in Bone Grafted Foot and Ankle Arthrodeses: A Retrospective Review," Second World Congress for Electricity and Magnetism in Biology and Medicine, 8–13 June 1997, Bologna, Italy.

T. Zizic, et al., "The Treatment of Rheumatoid Arthritis of the Hand with Pulsed Electrical Fields," Second World Congress for Electricity and Magnetism in Biology and Medicine, 8–13 June 1997, Bologna, Italy.

This double-blind, placebo-controlled study examined the effects of pulsed electrical fields administered over a period of 4 weeks in the treatment of arthritis of the hand. Results showed significant clinical improvement in patients receiving the therapy relative to controls.

V.D. Grigor'eva, et al., "Therapeutic Use of Physical Factors in Complex Therapy of Patients with Psoriatic Arthritis," *Vopr Kurortol Fizioter Lech Fiz Kult,* (6), 1995, pp. 48–51.

In this general review article on the treatment of patients with psoriatic arthritis with magnetic fields, the authors state that an alternating low-frequency magnetic field (30–40 mT) from such generators as "Polius-1" and "Polius-101" improves the clinical state of afflicted joints. Such treatments are normally carried out for 30 minutes per day over a period of 15 to 20 days.

B.Y. Drozdovski, et al., "Use of Magnetolaser Therapy with an AMLT-01 Apparatus in Complex Therapy for Rheumatoid Arthritis," *Fiz Med,* 4(1–2), 1994, pp. 101–102.

This study examined the effects of magnetolaser therapy either itself or in combination with conventional drugs in patients suffering from rheumatoid arthritis. Magnetolaser therapy involved the use of an AMLT-01 device and consisted of 6-minute exposures daily over a total of 14 days.

Results showed a marked improvement following the first 3 days of magnetolaser therapy, with the strongest positive effects experienced by patients characterized as suffering from mild to moderate levels of the disease. At the end of the magnetolaser therapy course, 90 percent of patients showed improvement.

E.A. Shlyapok, et al., "Use of Alternating Low-Frequency Magnetic Fields in Combination with Radon Baths for Treatment of Juvenile Rheumatoid Arthritis," *Vopr Kurortol Fizioter Lech Fiz Kult*, 4, 1992, pp. 13–17.

This study examined the effects of low-frequency magnetic fields (from a "Polius-1" device) in patients 7 to 14 years old suffering from juvenile rheumatoid arthritis. Treatment consisted of 10 daily exposures of 10 to 12 minutes each. Results showed beneficial effects in 58, 76, and 37 percent of patients in each of three experimental groups.

V.D. Grigor'eva, et al., "Therapeutic Application of Low-Frequency and Constant Magnetic Fields in Patients with Osteoarthritis Deformans and Rheumatoid Arthritis," *Vopr Kurortol Fizioter Lech Fiz Kult*, 4, 1980, pp. 29–35.

This study examined the effects of low-frequency and constant magnetic fields in patients suffering from rheumatoid arthritis and osteoarthrosis. Low-frequency magnetic fields were shown to produce beneficial effects in patients with both Stage I and II rheumatoid arthritis and with osteoarthrosis deformans, especially with respect to the wrists, knees, and ankles.

BLEPHARITIS (INFECTION OF THE EYELID)

V.A. Machekhin, et al., "A New Method for Treating Chronic Blepharitis Using Magnetic Compounds and an Alternating Magnetic Field," *Vestn Oftalmol,* 109(4), July–September 1993, pp. 16–18.

Results of this study indicated that the use of an alternating magnetic field in conjunction with a magnetic ointment containing reduced iron powder had beneficial effects in patients with chronic blepharitis.

BONE FRACTURES

V.A. Machekhin, et al., "A New Method for Treating Chronic Blepharitis Using Magnetic Compounds and an Alternating Magnetic Field," *Vestn Oftalmol,* 109(4), 1993, pp. 16–18.

C.A. Bassett, et al., "Treatment of Therapeutically Resistant Non-unions with Bone Grafts and Pulsing Electromagnetic Fields," *Journal of Bone Joint Surg,* 64(8), October 1982, pp. 1214–1220.

This study examined the effects of bone grafting and pulsed electromagnetic fields on a group of 83 adults with ununited fractures. Results showed a successful healing rate of 87 percent in the 38 patients originally treated with bone grafts and PEMF for ununited fractures with wide gaps, synovial pseudarthrosis, and malalignment. A healing rate of 93 percent was shown among the 45 patients who had initially been unsuccessfully treated with PEMF alone and had bone grafting and were retreated with pulsing electromagnetic fields.

C.A. Bassett, et al., "Treatment of Ununited Tibial Diaphyseal Fractures with Pulsing Electromagnetic Fields," *Journal of Bone Joint Surg*, 63(4), April 1981, pp. 511–23.

This study examined the effects of pulsing electromagnetic fields on 125 patients suffering from ununited fractures of the tibial diaphysis. Results showed a healing rate of 87 percent.

M.W. Meskens, et al., "Treatment of Delayed Union and Nonunion of the Tibia Pulsed Electromagnetic Fields. A Retrospective Follow-up," Bull Hosp Jt Dis Orthop Inst, 48(2), Fall 1988, pp. 170–175.

Results of this study showed treatment with pulsed electromagnetic fields resulted in an overall success rate of at least 75 percent in patients suffering from tibial lesions.

C.A. Bassett, "The Development and Application of Pulsed Electromagnetic Fields (PEMFs) for Ununited Fractures and Arthrodeses," *Clin Plast Surg*, 12(2), April 1985, pp. 259–277.

This review article makes the following observations with respect to the use of pulsed electromagnetic fields in treating ununited fractures, failed arthrodeses, and congenital pseudoarthroses. The treatment has been shown to be more than 90 percent effective in adult patients. In cases where union does not occur with PEMFs alone after approximately four months, PEMF treatment coupled with fresh bone grafts ensures a maximum failure rate of only 1 to 1.5 percent. For those with delayed union three to four months following fracture, PEMFs appear to be more successful than in patients treated with other conservative methods. For more serious conditions, including infected nonunions, multiple surgical failures, long-standing atrophic lesions, failed knee arthrodeses after removal of infected prostheses, and congenital pseudarthroses, PEMF treatment has exhibited success in most patients.

G.K. Frykman, et al., "Treatment of Nonunited Scaphoid Fractures Pulsed Electromagnetic Field and Cast," *Journal of Hand Surg,* 11(3), May 1986, pp. 344–349.

Results of this study found that 35 of 44 nonunited scaphoid fractures 6 months or older healed in a mean time of 4.3 months during pulsed electromagnetic field treatment using external coils and a thumb spica cast.

E. Betti, et al., "Effect of Electromagnetic Field Stimulation on Fractures of the Femoral Neck. A Prospective Randomized Double-Blind Study," Second World Congress for Electricity and Magnetism in Biology and Medicine, 8–13 June 1997, Bologna, Italy.

This double-blind, placebo-controlled study examined the effects of pulsed electromagnetic fields in femoral neck fracture patients undergoing conventional therapy. PEMF treatment was started within two weeks of fracture, and patients were instructed to make use of the electromagnetic device for 8 hours per day over a 90-day period. Results showed beneficial effects relative to controls after 18 months of follow-up.

V. Sollazzo, et al., "Effects of Pulsed Electromagnetic Fields (PEMF) on Human Osteoblast-Like Cells and Human Chondryocytes: An In Vitro Study," Second World Congress for Electricity and Magnetism in Biology and Medicine, 8–13 June 1997, Bologna, Italy.

J.T. Rya, et al., "Combine Magnetic Fields Stimulate Insulin-Like Growth Factor Production Potential Transcription Factor-Dependent Mechanism(s)," Second World Congress for Electricity and Magnetism in Biology and Medicine, 8–13 June 1997, Bologna, Italy.

C.A. Bassett, et al., "Pulsing Electromagnetic Field Treatment in Ununited Fractures and Failed Arthrodeses," *JAMA*, 247(5), February 5, 1982, pp. 623–628.

This review article on pulsing electromagnetic fields in the treatment of bone fracture observes that the surgically non-invasive outpatient method approved by the FDA in 1979 produced confirmed end results in 1007 ununited fractures and 71 failed arthrodeses, with an overall success rate at Columbia-Presbyterian Medical Center of 81 percent; an international success rate of 79 percent, and a success rate with other patients in the United States of 76 percent.

G.C. Traina, "Electromagnetic Field Stimulation of Osteotomies," Second World Congress for Electricity and Magnetism in Biology and Medicine, 8–13 June 1997, Bologna, Italy.

J. Nepola, et al., "Effect of Exposure Time on Stimulation of Healing in the Rabbit Tibial Osteotomy Model, a Time Varying Pulsed Electromagnetic Field, and a Combined Magnetic Field," Second World Congress for Electricity and Magnetism in Biology and Medicine, 8–13 June 1997, Bologna, Italy.

G. Borsalino, et al., "Electrical Stimulation of Human Femoral Intertrochanteric Osteotomies. Double-Blind Study," *Clin Orthop*, (237), December 1988, pp. 256–263.

Results of this double-blind study showed significant healing effects of low-frequency pulsing electromagnetic fields in patients treated with femoral intertrochanteric osteotomy for hip degenerative arthritis.

M. Marcer, et al., "Results of Pulsed Electromagnetic Fields (PEMFs) in Ununited Fractures after External Skeletal Fixation," *Clin Orthop*, (190), November 1984, pp. 260–265.

In this study, 147 patients with fractures of the tibia, femur, and humerus who had failed to benefit from surgery received treatment with external skeletal fixation in situ and pulsed electromagnetic fields. Results indicated an overall success rate of 73 percent. Femur union was seen in 81 percent and tibia union in 75 percent.

O. Wahlstrom, "Stimulation of Fracture Healing with Electromagnetic Fields of Extremely Low Frequency (EMF of ELF)," *Clin Orthop*, (186), June 1984, pp. 293–301.

This study examined the effects of extremely low frequency electromagnetic fields (1–1000 Hz, 4 gauss) on new bone fractures of female patients. Results led the authors to suggest that EMF treatment accelerates the early stages of fracture healing.

A.W. Dunn & G.A. Rush, 3d, "Electrical Stimulation in Treatment of Delayed Union and Nonunion of Fractures and Osteotomies," *Southern Medical Journal*, 77(12), December 1984, pp. 1530–1534.

G. Fontanesi, et al., "Slow Healing Fractures: Can They be Prevented? (Results of Electrical Stimulation in Fibular Osteotomies in Rats and in Diaphyseal Fractures of the Tibia in Humans)," *Italian Journal of Orthop Traumatol*, 12(3), September 1986, pp. 371–385.

This study examined the preventive effects of low-frequency pulsing electromagnetic fields against delayed union in rat fibular osteotomies and diaphyseal tibia fractures in humans. Results indicated such treatment modulated and accelerated fracture union in both groups.

F. Rajewski & W. Marciniak, "Use of Magnetotherapy for Treatment of Bone Malunion in Limb Lengthening. Preliminary Report," *Chir Narzadow Ruchu Ortop Pol*, 57(1–3), 1992, pp. 247–249.

This article discusses the cases of two children with bone malunion following lengthening of congenitally shortened lower legs. Pulsed sinusoidal magnetic field treatment was beneficial for both patients.

R.B. Simonis, et al., "The Treatment of Non-union Pulsed Electromagnetic Fields Combined with a Denham External Fixator," *Injury*, 15(4), January 1984, pp. 255–260.

Results of this study showed that 13 of 15 cases of long-bone nonunion treated with pulsed electromagnetic fields in combination with Denham external fixator united within several months.

L. Sedel, et al., "Acceleration of Repair of Non-unions Electromagnetic Fields," *Rev Chir Orthop Reparatrice Appar Mot*, 67(1), 1981, pp. 11–23.

Results of this study found electromagnetic field stimulation to be an effective treatment for nonunion among a group of 37 French patients.

J.C. Mulier & F. Spaas, "Out-patient Treatment of Surgically Resistant Non-unions Induced Pulsing Current—Clinical Results," *Arch Orthop Trauma Surg*, 97(4), 1980, pp. 293–297.

Results of this study found treatment induced pulsing to be beneficial in patients suffering from nonunions unresponsive to surgery.

C.A. Bassett, "Conversations with C. Andrew L. Bassett, M.D. Pulsed Electromagnetic Fields. A Noninvasive Therapeutic Modality for Fracture Nonunion (Interview)," *Orthop. Review*, 15(12), 1986, pp. 781–795.

In this interview with Dr. C. Andrew L. Bassett, a physician researching the use of pulsed electromagnetic fields for the past 30 years at Columbia University's Orthopedic Research Lab, Dr. Bassett notes that approximately 10,000 of the 12,000-plus orthopedic surgeons in the United States have used pulsed electromagnetic fields on at least one patient. Many such surgeons have incorporated the therapy on a more regular basis. He estimates that a total of at least 65,000 patients nationwide have received the treatment, with a probable success rate of between 80 and 90 percent. Use of the treatment has been primarily in patients suffering from nonunited fractures, fusion failures, and pseudoarthrosis.

B.T. O'Connor, "Treatment of Surgically Resistant Nonunions with Pulsed Electromagnetic Fields," *Reconstr Surg Traumatology*, 19, 1985, pp. 123–132.

Results of this study showed pulsed electromagnetic fields to have beneficial healing effects in patients suffering from difficult-to-treat and surgically resistant bone nonunions.

A. Bassett, "Therapeutic Uses of Electric and Magnetic Fields in Orthopedics," in D.O. Carpenter & S. Ayrapetyan, (eds.), *Biological Effects of Electric and Magnetic Fields. Volume II: Beneficial and Harmful Effects*, San Diego: Academic Press, 1994, pp. 13–48.

This review article notes that the use of pulsed electromagnetic fields began in 1974, and that 250,000 nonunion patients have received the treatment since. The author argues that success rates are comparable to those of bone grafting, and that PEMF treatment is more cost-effective and free of side effects. The FDA approved PEMF use in 1982, although it remains widely unused due to physician misunderstanding and lack of knowledge concerning the treatment.

A.A. Goldberg, "Computer Analysis of Data on More than 11,000 Cases of Ununited Fracture Submitted for Treatment with Pulsing Electromagnetic Fields," Bioelectrical Repair and Growth Society, Second Annual Meeting, 20–22 September 1982, Oxford, UK, p. 61.

This 7-year study examined data on more than 11,000 cases of nonunions treated with pulsed electromagnetic fields for up to 10 to 12 hours per day. Results indicated an overall success rate of 75 percent.

O. Wahlstrom, "Electromagnetic Fields Used in the Treatment of Fresh Fractures of the Radius," Bioelectrical Repair and Growth Society, Second Annual Meeting, 20–22 September 1982, Oxford, UK, p. 26.

This study examined the effects of low-frequency electromagnetic fields (1-1000 Hz) on middle-aged female patients suffering from fresh radius fractures. Results showed significant increases in scintimetric activity surrounding the fracture area after two weeks of EMF treatment relative to controls.

G.B. Gromak & G.A. Lacis, "Evaluations of the Efficacy of Using a Constant Magnetic Field in Treatment of Patients with Traumas," in I. Detlav, (ed.), Electromagnetic Therapy of Injuries and Diseases of the Support-Motor Apparatus. International Collection of Papers, Riga, Latvia: Riga Medical Institute, 1987, pp. 88–95.

This study examined the effects of constant magnetic fields in patients suffering from fractures. Results showed that magnetic exposure reduced pain and the onset of edema shortly after trauma. Where edema was already present, the treatment exhibited marked anti-inflammatory effects. The strongest beneficial effects occurred in patients suffering from fractures of the ankle joints.

A.F. Lynch & P. MacAuley, "Treatment of Bone Non-Union Electromagnetic Therapy," *Ir Journal of Med Sci*, 154(4), 1985, pp. 153–155.

Results of this study found that 10 hours per day of electromagnetic stimulation (1.0–1.5 mV) produced complete union in 23 of 26 patients receiving the treatment for non-joined fractures.

C.A.L. Bassett, "Historical Overview of PEM-Assisted Bone and Tissue Healing," Bioelectromagnetics Society, 10th Annual Meeting, 19–24 June 1988, Stamford, CT, p. 19.

This review article looks at the history of pulsed electromagnetic fields as a means of bone repair. The author argues that success rates have been either superior or equivalent to those of surgery, with PEMF free of side effects and risk.

BRONCHITIS

V.M. Iurlov, et al., "The Efficacy of the Use of Low-Frequency Electromagnetic Fields in Chronic Bronchitis," *Voen Med Zh*, 3, 1989, pp. 35–36.

Results of this double-blind, placebo-controlled study indicated that both low-frequency electromagnetic field treatment and treatment with pulsed electromagnetic fields proved effective in patients suffering from chronic bronchitis when coupled with standard drug therapies. Magnetic field treatment consisted of a total of 15 15–20-minute daily exposures.

CANCER

R.R. Raylman, et al., "Exposure to Strong Static Magnetic Field Slows the Growth of Human Cancer Cells in Vitro," *Bioelectromagnetics*, 17(5), 1996, pp. 358–363.

Results of this study found that prolonged exposure to a 7-tesla uniform static magnetic field for a period of 64 hours inhibited growth of three human tumor cell lines in vitro.

N.G. Bakhmutskii, et al., "The Assessment of the Efficacy of the Effect of a Rotational Magnetic Field on the Course of the Tumor Process in Patients with Generalized Breast Cancer," *Sov Med,* (7), 1991, pp. 25–27.

This study examined the effects of a rotational magnetic field on a group of 51 breast cancer patients. Results showed a significant positive response in 27 of them.

N.G. Bakhmutskii, et al., "The Growth Dynamics of Walker Carcinosarcoma During Exposure to a Magnetic Eddy Field," *Vopr Onkol,* 37(6), 1991, pp. 705–708.

Results of this study indicated that exposure to a rotational magnetic field inhibited Walker's carcinoma tumor growth as much as 90 percent in some cases.

Y. Omote, "An Experimental Attempt to Potentiate Therapeutic Effects of Combined Use of Pulsing Magnetic Fields and Antitumor Agents," *Nippon Geka Gakkai Zasshi,* 89(8), August 1988, pp. 1155–1166.

Results of this study indicated that pulsed magnetic field stimulation increased the incorporation of antitumor agents into cells, and thus increased antitumor activity shifting the cell cycle to a proliferative from a nonproliferative phase.

L.S. Ogorodnikova, et al., "Morphological Criteria of Lung Cancer Regression Under the Effect of Magnetotherapy," *Vopr Onkol,* 26(1), 1980, pp. 28–34.

Results of this study found that 20–30 sessions of magnetotherapy administered preoperatively exhibited antitumor effects in patients suffering from lung cancer.

C.K. Chou, et al., "Development of Electrochemical Treatment at the City of Hope," Second World Congress for Electricity and Magnetism in Biology and Medicine, 8–13 June 1997, Bologna, Italy.

S. Yunqin, et al., "Electrochemical Therapy in the Treatment of Malignant Tumours on the Body Surface," *European Journal of Surgery,* 160(574 Suppl), 1994, pp. 41–43.

D.V. Miasoedov, et al., "Experience with the Use of Microwave Resonance Therapy as a Modifying Factor in Oncological Therapy," *Abstracts of the First All-Union Symposium with International Participation,* May 10–13, 1989, Kiev, Ukraine, pp. 313–315.

This study examined the effects of microwave resonance therapy (MRT) in patients suffering from various forms of cancer. Results showed that MRT treatment prior to surgery reduced the spread of cancer-associated conditions and reduced the risk associated with surgery in 87 percent of patients. MRT applied postoperatively had beneficial effects in 68 percent.

U. Randoll & R.M. Pangan, "The Role of Complex Biophysical-Chemical Therapies for Cancer," *Bioelectrochem Bioenerg,* 27(3), 1992, pp. 341–346.

Results of this study proved that the combination of weak pulsed electromagnetic fields with antioxidant supplementation is beneficial in the treatment of patients suffering from tongue cancer, improving speech, pain control, and tolerance to chemotherapy.

V.G. Andreev, et al., "Radiomodifying Effect of a Constant Magnetic Field in Radiation Therapy of Patients with Cancer of the Throat," *Fizicheskaia Meditzina*, 4(1–2), 1994, p. 92.

Results of this controlled study indicated that treatment with a constant magnetic field significantly improved long-term (3-year) survival time in patients undergoing radiation therapy for cancer of the throat. Constant magnetic field therapy consisted of the application of 300 mT for 30 minutes to tumor and metastasizing regions immediately prior to each irradiation.

V. Smirnova, "Anti-Tumorigenic Action of an Eddy Magnetic Field," *Vrach*, 2, 1994, pp. 25–26.

Results of this Russian study indicated that the use of whole body eddy magnetic fields, coupled with more conventional cancer therapies (including magnetotherapy) is effective in the treatment of patients suffering from a variety of different malignancies.

N.G. Bakhmutskii, et al., "A Case of Successful Treatment of a Patient with Breast Cancer Using a Rotating Electromagnetic Field," *Soviet Medicine*, 8, 1991, pp. 86–87.

This article reports on the case of a 48-year-old-woman with breast cancer who was treated successfully with magnetotherapy. Infiltration showed a marked decrease following 30 whole body exposures to an eddy magnetic field for 60 minutes. One metastatic node disappeared while the size of others was reduced following 60 such exposures. A total regression of tumor and metastases was seen following the completion of a course of 110 exposures.

V.A. Lubennikov, et al., "First Experience in Using a Whole-Body Magnetic Field Exposure in Treating Cancer Patients," *Vopr Onkol,* 41(2), 1995, pp. 140–141.

This study examined the effects of whole body magnetic fields (16.5–35 G, 50–165 Hz) on patients suffering from different forms of cancer. Treatment consisted of 15 cycles, each 1–20 minutes in duration, and was coupled with more traditional cancer therapies. Results showed that the magnetotherapy had overall beneficial effects, particularly with respect to improved immune status and postoperative recovery.

I. Rodin, et al., "Use of Low-Intensity Eddy Magnetic Field in the Treatment of Patients with Skin Lymphomas," *Voen Med Zh,* 317(12), 1996, pp. 32–34.

CARDIOVASCULAR/CORONARY HEART DISEASE

M.A. Dudchenko, et al., "The Effect of Combined Treatment with the Use of Magnetotherapy on the Systemic Hemodynamics of Patients with Ischemic Heart Disease and Spinal Osteochondrosis," *Lik Sprava,* (5), May 1992, pp. 40–43.

Results of this study found that the addition of magnetotherapy to the treatment of patients suffering from ischemic heart disease and osteochondrosis led to clinical improvements.

E.M. Vasil'eva, et al., "The Effect of a Low-frequency Magnetic Field on Erythrocyte Membrane Function and on the Prostanoid Level in the Blood Plasma of Children with Parasystolic Arrhythmia," *Vopr Kurortol Fizioter Lech Fiz Kult*, (2), March–April 1994, pp. 18–20.

Results of this study involving 23 parasystolic children found that low-frequency magnetic field exposure improved humoral and cellular processes involved in the regulation of cardiac rhythm.

Y.B. Kirillov, et al., "Magnetotherapy in Obliterating Vascular Diseases of the Lower Extremities," *Vopr Kurortol Fizioter Lech Fiz Kult*, (3), May–June 1992, pp. 14–17.

The authors of this study report on their development of a polymagnetic system called Avrora-MK-01 used to administer impulse magnetic fields to diseases of the leg vessels. Results indicated positive effects on peripheral capillaries in 75–82 percent of patients receiving the treatment at a pre-gangrene stage.

O.M. Konova & M.A. Khan, "The Effect of a Low-frequency Alternating Magnetic Field on the Autonomic Nervous System in Children with Primary Arterial Hypertension," *Vopr Kurortol Fizioter Lech Fiz Kult*, (2), March–April, 1996, pp. 8–10.

Results of this study showed exposure to low-frequency alternating magnetic fields had beneficial effects in children with primary arterial hypertension, as seen in the attenuation of sympathetic and vagotonic symptoms.

V.S. Zadionchenko, et al., "Prognostic Criteria of the Efficacy of Magnetic and Magnetic-laser Therapy in Patients with the Initial Stages of Hypertension," *Vopr Kurortol Fizioter Lech Fiz Kult,* (1), January–February 1997, pp. 8–11.

This study demonstrated that traveling pulsed magnetic field and magnetic laser treatment produced beneficial effects in patients suffering from the initial stages of essential hypertension.

R.T. Gordon & D. Gordon, "Selective Resolution of Plaques and Treatment of Atherosclerosis Biophysical Alteration of "Cellular" and "Intracellular" Properties," *Medical Hypotheses,* 7(2), February 1981, pp. 217–229.

In this article, the authors propose a new approach to treating atherosclerosis through the alteration of biophysical properties both intracellularly and extracellularly. Citing their own preliminary data, they suggest atherosclerotic lesions might be selectively resolved without harming normal blood vessels, allowing the lesions to take up the magnetically excitable submicron particles and then applying an external alternating electromagnetic field.

S.G. Ivanov, et al., "The Magnetotherapy of Hypertension Patients," *Ter Arkh,* 62(9), 1990, pp. 71–74.

This study examined the effects of constant MKM2-1 magnets on essential hypertension patients. Results indicated the treatment decreased arterial pressure in Stage II patients, with magnetotherapy being shown to produce beneficial effects on the central hemodynamics and microcirculation.

R. Cadossi, "Protective Effect of Electromagnetic Field Exposure on Acute Soft Tissue Ischaemic Injury," Second World Congress for Electricity and Magnetism in Biology and Medicine, 8–13 June 1997, Bologna, Italy.

Results from several recent studies conducted by the author are reviewed. Conclusions are that pulsed electromagnetic fields exhibit protective effects against necrosis from acute ischemia in rats, cerebral infarcts in rabbits, and myocardium infarcts in rats.

I.E. Ganelina, et al., "Electromagnetic Radiation of Extremely High Frequencies in Complex Therapy for Severe Stenocardia," *Millimetrovie Volni v Biologii I Meditcine*, (4), 1994, pp. 17–21.

This study examined the effects of extremely high frequency electromagnetic radiation (EHF EMR) in 93 patients suffering ischemic heart disease. EHF treatment consisted of 10 to 15 exposures of the lower end of the sternum from a 'Yav'-1-7,1 device. Treatment was performed five times weekly for a total of 30 minutes per day, with drug therapy being maintained during this period. Positive results tended to occur after 5 to 6 treatment sessions, with a good or satisfactory response being reported in 82 of 93 patients, and lasting as long as 11 months after hospital release.

T.V. Golovacheva, "EHF Therapy in Complex Treatment of Cardiovascular Diseases," *Millimeter Waves in Medicine and Biology*, 10th Russian Symposium with International Participation, April 24–26, 1995, Moscow, Russia, pp. 29–31.

V.V. Orzeshkovskii, et al., "Clinical Application of Electromagnetic Fields," in I.G. Akoevs & V.V. Tiazhelov, (eds.), *Topics of Experimental and Applied Bioelectromagnetics. A Collection of Research Papers*, Puschcino, USSR, USSR Academy of Sciences, Biological Sciences Research Center, 1983, pp. 139–147.

This review article concerning the clinical application of electromagnetic fields notes that microwave therapy has been shown to improve local circulation and vascular tone, increase the volume of functional capillaries, lower hypertension, stimulate protein and carbohydrate metabolism, stimulate the pituitary-adrenal system, produce anti-inflammatory effects, and improve digestive organ function. Studies have shown decimeter wave therapy capable of stimulating the secretory function of the stomach, as well as blood circulation, respiratory function, and the immune system. Side effects have been reported in both human and animal studies.

N.N. Naumcheva, "Effect of Millimeter Waves on Ischemic Heart Disease Patients," *Millimetrovie Volni v Biologii I Meditcine*, (3), 1994, pp. 62–67.

In this study, 30 myocardial infarction patients received millimeter-wave (MW) therapy in the form of 10 exposures of 30 minutes per day, with a 2-day interruption after the fifth exposure. Patients continued conventional drug treatment during the MW therapy period. Better results were seen in those patients exposed to the MW therapy relative to an equal number of patients receiving conventional treatment only.

A.P. Dovganiuk & A.A. Minenkov, "The Use of Physical Factors in Treating Chronic Arterial Insufficiency of the Lower Limbs," *Vopr Kurortol Fizioter Lech Fiz Kult*, (5), 1996, pp. 7–9.

This study examined the effects of millimeter wave therapy in approximately 450 patients suffering from a variety of diseases, including those of the musculoskeletal, digestive, pulmonary, and nervous systems. Treatment consisted of 25–30 minutes per day using the "Porog-1" apparatus and generally lasted for a period of up to 10 days. Results showed positive effects in over 87 percent of the patients.

V.V. Orzheshovski, et al., "Efficacy of Decimeter-Band Waves and Magnetophore Therapy in Patients with Hypertension," *Vrach Delo*, (1), 1982, pp. 65–67.

Results of this study found that the use of magnetophore therapy (constant magnets applied to adrenal regions 10 hours per day for 15 days) significantly improved symptoms associated with hypertension in about 35 percent of patients studied, with mild improvement seen in 30 percent, and no improvement in 35 percent. Patients receiving decimeter-band waves (460 MHz, field intensity of 35–45 W, for 10–15 minutes per day for a total of 15 days) experienced similar results.

L.L. Orlov, et al., "Indications for Using a New Mag-
netotherapeutic Method in Arterial Hypertension," *Soviet
Medicine*, (8), 1991, pp. 23–24.

Results of this placebo-controlled study demonstrated a 76
percent effectiveness rate for running impulse magnetic field
therapy in a group of arterial hypertensive patients. Treatment consisted of two 25-minute exposures per day over a
period of 10–20 total exposures, at frequencies of 10 or 100
Hz and magnetic field intensity of 3 or 10 mT.

V.V. Orzheshkovskii, et al., "The Treatment of Hypertension Patients with Electromagnetic and Magnetic Fields,"
Vrach Delo, (10), 1991, pp. 81–82.

I.G. Alizade, et al., "Magnetic Treatment of Autologous
Blood in the Combined Therapy of Hypertensive Patients,"
Vopr Kurortol Fizioter Lech Fiz Kult, (1), 1994, pp. 32–33.

This study examined the efficacy of the reinfusion of autologous blood following magnetic field exposure in hypertensive patients. Positive effects were found in 92 percent of
patients receiving the treatment.

E.V. Rolovlev, "Treatment of Essential Hypertension Patients by an Alternating Magnetic Field Puncture," All-
Union Symposium: Laser and Magnetic Therapy in
Experimental and Clinical Studies, June 16–18, 1993, Ob-
ninsk, Kaluga Region, Russia, pp. 221–223.

This double-blind, placebo-controlled study examined the
effects of magnetotherapy in patients suffering from first- or

second-stage hypertension. A magnetic field of 50 Hz, 15–25 mT was applied to acupuncture points He-Gu and Shen'-Men for 15–20 seconds per day for a total of 9–10 days. Results: The treatment improved headaches in 88 percent of patients, dizziness in 89 percent, and irritability in 88 percent. In general, 95 percent of hypertensive patients experienced beneficial effects from the treatment, and the morbidity rate decreased twofold following one course extended over a period of 5–6 months.

I.N. Danilova & E.M. Orekhova, "Application of Sinusoidally-Modulated Currents in the Electrosleep Therapeutic Procedure," *Vopr Kurortol Fizioter Lech Fiz Kult,* (6), 1989, pp. 9–13.

S.G. Ivanov, et al., "Use of Magnetic Fields in the Treatment of Hypertensive Disease," *Vopr Kurortol Fizioter Lech Fiz Kult,* (3), 1993, pp. 67–69.

This placebo-controlled study examined the effects of constant and of running magnetic fields in patients suffering from Stage II hypertension. Results found that constant magnetic fields exhibited benefits in 68 percent of patients treated, and running magnetic fields were helpful in 78 percent. Only 30 percent of controls showed improvement. Constant magnetic field treatment consisted of constant magnets applied to the inner side of the wrist on each hand for 35–40 minutes daily over a period of 7–10 days. Running magnetic field treatment involved the use of a "Alimp-1" apparatus for 20 minutes per day for a total of 12–15 days.

S.G. Ivanov, "The Comparative Efficacy of Nondrug and Drug Methods of Treating Hypertension," *Ter Arkh*, 65(1), 1993, pp. 44–49.

This double-blind, placebo-controlled study found that magnetotherapy was effective in the treatment of symptoms associated with Stage II hypertension, such as headache, dizziness, and cardiodynia. The therapy consisted of permanent circular magnets (16 mT) applied to the inner forearm for 30–45 minutes per day over a period of 10 sessions.

T.A. Kniazeva & R. Arutiunian, "The Effect of Low-Frequency Magnetic Field and General Iodobromide Baths with the Presence of Molecular Iodine on the Blood Coagulation Processes and the Central Hemodynamics of Patients after an Aortocoronary passs," *Vopr Kurortol Fizioter Lech Fiz Kult*, 4, 1990, pp. 11–15.

L.N. Budkar, et al., "Magnetolaser Therapy in Treatment of Ischemic Heart Disease and Heart Rhythm Disorders," *Doktor Lending*, 4(13), 1996, pp. 10–13.

L.L. Orlov, et al., "Effect of a Running Pulse Magnetic Field on Some Humoral Indices and Physical Capacity in Patients with Neurocirculatory Hypo- and Hypertension," *Biofizika*, 41(4), 1996, pp. 944–948.

This controlled study examined the effects of magnetotherapy in patients suffering from neurocirculatory hypotension (low blood pressure) or hypertension (high blood pressure). Treatment consisted of a running pulsed magnetic field generated by an "ALIMP" device (0.5 mT, 300 Hz) administered for 20 minutes per day over a course of 10 days. Patients suffering from hypotension did not benefit significantly from the magnetotherapy. Hypertension patients, however, showed a marked improvement with respect to symptoms including headache, chest pain, extremity numbness, abnormal systolic and diastolic blood pressure, and work capacity.

T.A. Kniazeva, "The Efficacy of Low-Intensity Exposures in Hypertension," *Vopr Kurortol Fizioter Lech Fiz Kult*, 1, 1994, pp. 8–9.

This double-blind, placebo-controlled study found that low-frequency, low-intensity electrostatic fields (40–62 Hz) administered for 12–14 minutes per day helped normalize blood pressure in patients suffering from hypertension.

A.G. Kakulia, "The Use of Sonic Band Magnetic Fields in Various Diseases," *Vopr Kurortol Fizioter Lech Fiz Kult*, 3, 1982, pp. 18–21.

This study examined the effects of low-frequency alternating magnetic fields in patients suffering from arteriosclerosis or osteoarthrosis deformans. Treatment involved 10–15 minute daily leg exposures over a total of 15 days. Results showed the treatment to be effective in 80 percent of arteriosclerosis patients and 70 percent of those with osteoarthrosis deformans.

S.S. Gabrielian, et al., "Use of Low-Frequency Magnetic Fields in the Treatment of Patients with Atherosclerotic Encephalopathy," *Vopr Kurortol Fizioter Lech Fiz Kult*, 3, 1987, pp. 36–39.

This study examined the effects of low-frequency magnetic fields (25 mT) in patients suffering atherosclerotic encephalopathy. Treatment involved 10–15 minute daily exposures over a total of 10–15 applications. Results showed clinical improvements with respect to chest pain, vertigo, headache, and other symptoms.

CHRONIC VENOUS INSUFFICIENCY

N.A. Temur'iants, et al., "Use of Millimeter-Wave Therapy for Increasing of Nonspecific Resistivity in Children Suffering from Frequent and Long-Lasting Catarrhal Diseases," *Millimetrovie Volni v Biologii I Meditcine*, 3, 1994, pp. 85–88.

E.I. Pasynkov, et al., "Therapeutic Use of Alternating Magnetic Field in the Treatment of Patients with Chronic Diseases of the Veins of the Lower Limbs," *Vopr Kurortol Fizioter Lech Fiz Kult*, 5, 1976, pp. 16–19.

This study examined the effects of alternating magnetic fields (15–20 minutes per day over a period of 20 days) in patients suffering from chronic venous insufficiency, varicose veins, and trophic shin ulcers. Results showed good effects in 236 of the 271 patients receiving the treatment. Thirty-four patients reported satisfactory effects. Only one patient experienced no effects.

A.P. Dovganiuk, "Balneologic and Physical Therapy of Chronic Venous Insufficiency of Extremities," *Vopr Kurortol Fizioter Lech Fiz Kult*, 2, 1995, pp. 48–49.

This review article notes that magnetotherapy in a variety of forms has been successfully used in the treatment of chronic venous insufficiency and is a commonly used physical therapy for the condition.

Y.B. Kirillov, et al., "Magnetotherapy for Obliterative Disease of the Vessels of the Legs," *Vopr Kurortol Fizioter Lech Fiz Kult*, 3, 1992, pp. 14–17.

This study examined the effects of running impulse magnetic fields in patients suffering from vessel obliteration diseases of the legs. Treatment consisted of 15–20 whole body exposures (0.5-5 mT, 1–2 Hz) lasting 15–20 minutes each. Results showed treatment led to a significant reduction in the number of patients experiencing leg pain while at rest. Among patients previously unable to walk a 500-m distance, 52 percent were able to complete the distance following treatment. Circulation improved in 75–82 percent of patients.

E.N. Grebnev & A.V. Shumskii, "Immunocorrective Therapy in the Treatment of Chronic Herpetic Stomatitis Using Magnetic Autohemotherapy," *Stomatologiia* (Mosk), 74(2), 1995, pp. 37–39.

R.G. Schwartz, "Electric Sympathetic Block: An Advanced Clinical Technique for the Treatment of Complex Acute Chronic Pain," Second World Congress for Electricity and

Magnetism in Biology and Medicine, 8–13 June 1997, Bologna, Italy.

N.V. Ordzhonikidze, et al., "Experimental Validation of the Efficacy of Laser-magnetic Therapy for Chronic Placental Insufficiency," *Akush Ginekol* (Mosk), (1), 1994, pp. 18–21.

T.N. Leont'eva, "Ultrasonic Ethmoidotomy Combined with Intracavitary Magnetotherapy in Chronic Polypous Ethmoiditis," *Vestn Otorinolaringol,* (4), July–August 1990, pp. 38–41.

S.P. Seregin & A.V. Panov, "The Correction of Prostatic Hemodynamics in Chronic Prostatitis," *Vopr Kurortol Fizioter Lech Fiz Kult,* (2), March–April 1997, pp. 20–21.

A.D. Deineka & A.M. Pozdniakov, "Magnetolaser Therapy of Constitutional Hyperbilrubinemia," *Fiz Med,* 4(1–2), 1994, pp. 104–105.

A.A. Verzin, "Action of Gentamycin Against a Background of Magnetotherapy of the Anterior Chamber in a Traumatic Infected Erosion of the Cornea," *Antibiotiki,* 27(10), October 1982, pp. 774–775.

M.A. Darendeliler, et al., "Light Maxillary Expansion Forces with the Magnetic Expansion Device. A Preliminary Investigation," *European Journal of Orthod,* 16(6), December 1994, pp. 479–490.

A. Breunig & T. Rakosi, "The Treatment of Open Bite Using Magnets," *Fortschr Kieferorthop*, 53(3), June 1992, pp. 179–186.

F.G. Sander & A. Wichelhaus, "Can Magnets or Additional Intermaxillary Forces Improve the Mode of Action of Jumping-the-bite Plates?" *Fortschr Kieferorthop*, 55(6), December 1994, pp. 279–289.

D. Zaffe, et al., "PEMFS Improve Bone Adaptation in Orthodontically Treated Rabbits," Second World Congress for Electricity and Magnetism in Biology and Medicine, 8–13 June 1997, Bologna, Italy.

DENTAL PROBLEMS

V.E. Kriokshina, et al., "Use of Micromagnets in Stomatology," *Magnitologiia*, (1), 1991, pp. 17–20.

This placebo-controlled study examined the effects of micromagnets in the treatment of periodontal disease. Micromagnets were attached to the skin over areas of inflammation for a period ranging from 1 to 8 days, with the number of magnets used at once varying from 1 to 6. The course of treatment lasted as long as 4 weeks. Results indicated that patients receiving the micromagnet therapy experienced earlier and more trouble-free recoveries following oral surgery, as well as less pain relative to controls.

L.C. Rhodes, "The Adjunctive Utilization of Diapulse Therapy (Pulsed High Peak Power Electromagnetic Energy) in Accelerating Tissue Healing in Oral Surgery," *Q National Dental Association*, 40(1), 1981, pp. 4–11.

This controlled study examined the effects of adjunctive Diapulse electromagnetic therapy on oral surgery recovery. Patients received the therapy once per day beginning between 3 to 5 days prior to oral surgery. Therapy was maintained until the point of hospital release. Results found the therapy produced significant healing relative to controls, who received conventional treatment only.

V. Hillier-Kolarov & N. Pekaric-Nadj, "PEMF Therapy as an Additional Therapy for Oral Diseases," European Bioelectromagnetics Association, 1st Congress, 23–25 January 1992, Brussels, Belgium.

This study found that patients suffering from various oral diseases experienced more rapid healing when treated with both conventional therapies and 30 minutes per day of pulsed electromagnetic fields (5 mT, 30 Hz), as opposed to conventional therapies alone.

A.A. Kunin, et al., "Magnetolaser Therapy in Complex Treatment of Periodontal Diseases," *Fiz Med*, 4(1–2), 1994, pp. 103–104.

DEPRESSION

M.T. Kirkcaldie, et al., Transcranial Magnetic Stimulation as Therapy for Depression and Other Disorders," *Aust N Z J Psychiatry*, 31(2), April 1997, pp. 264–272.

This review article examined the literature concerning the use of transcranial magnetic stimulation in the treatment of depression. Results showed the high-frequency, repetitive transcranial magnetic stimulation treatment to be an effective, side-effect-free therapy for depression that may hold promise for treating related psychiatric disorders as well.

R. Sandyk, et al., "Magnetic Felds and Seasonality of Affective Illness: Implications for Therapy," *International Journal of Neurosci,* 58(3–4), June 1991, pp. 261–267.

Noting that there is good reason to believe the pineal gland is a magnetosensitive system and that application of magnetic fields in experimental animals has a similar effect to that of acute exposure to light with respect to melatonin secretion, the authors propose that magnetic treatment could be a beneficial new therapy for winter depression in humans.

C. Haag, et al., "Transcranial Magnetic Stimulation. A Diagnostic Means from Neurology as Therapy in Psychiatry?" *Nervenarzt,* 68(3), March 1997, pp. 274–278.

This review article notes that transcranial magnetic stimulation has been shown to elicit antidepressant effects, electrically stimulating deep regions of the brain.

T. Zyss, "Will Electroconvulsive Therapy Induce Seizures: Magnetic Brain Stimulation as Hypothesis of a New Psychiatric Therapy," *Psychiatr Pol,* 26(6), November–December 1992, pp. 531–541.

In this theoretical paper, the author argues that deep, low-rate transcranial magnetic stimulation can produce therapeutic effects equivalent to those of electroconvulsive therapy but without the dangerous side effects.

G.V. Morozov, et al., "Extremely-High Frequency Electromagnetic Radiation in the Treatment of Neurotic Depression in Women," Millimeter Waves in Medicine and Biology. Digest of Papers of the 10th Russian Symposium with International Participation, April 24–26, 1995, Moscow, Russia, pp. 49–51.

G.V. Morozov, et al., "Treatment of Neurotic Depression with a Help of Extremely High Frequency Electromagnetic Radiation," Zh Nevropatol Psikhiatr Im S S Korsakova, 96(6), 1996, pp. 28–31.

This study examined the effects of millimeter wave (MW) therapy as a supplemental treatment in patients suffering from various types of depression. MW therapy involved the use of a "Yav'-1" apparatus (5.6 mm wavelength, 53 GHz), and consisted of up to 60 minutes of exposure per day, 2 to 3 times per week, for a total of as many as 15 exposures. Results showed that combined MW/conventional treatment produced a complete recovery in over 50 percent of cases studied, a significant improvement in 41 percent, and some improvement in 8 percent. Recovery rates among controls (conventional treatment only) were 4, 48, and 41 percent, respectively.

A. Conca, et al., "Transcranial Magnetic Stimulation: A Novel Antidepressive Strategy?" *Neuropsychobiology*, 34(4), 1996, pp. 204–207.

Results of this study led researchers to conclude that patients suffering from major depression experienced a significant reduction of depressive symptoms following treatment with transcranial magnetic stimulation coupled with standard medication relative to patients taking the medicine. This was true after just three TMS treatments.

DERMATITIS

V.P. Adaskevich, "Effectiveness of the Use of Millimeter-Range Electromagnetic Radiation in Complex Treatment of Atopic Dermatitis Patients," *Millimetrovie Volni v Biologii I Meditcine*, (3), 1994, pp. 78–81.

This study examined the effects of conventional treatments combined with millimeter wave (MW) therapy (54- to 70-GHz frequency, 8–15 daily exposures of 15–30 minutes each) on patients suffering from atopic dermatitis. Results indicated that the MW therapy was well tolerated by all patients, with the rash generally regressing after 7–8 exposures. Marked recovery was seen among 78 percent of patients receiving the combination treatments. Two-year follow-up showed a 23 percent relapse rate among combination patients, compared to 54 percent among controls.

DIABETES

I.B. Kirillovm, et al., "Magnetotherapy in the Comprehensive Treatment of Vascular Complications of Diabetes Mellitus," *Klin Med,* 74(5), 1996, pp. 39–41.

In this study, 320 diabetics received impulsed magnetic field treatment while 100 diabetics (controls) received conservative therapy alone. Results showed beneficial effects with respect to vascular complications in 74 percent of the patients receiving magnetotherapy combined with conservative methods, compared to a 28 percent effectiveness rate among controls.

M.I. Shved & A.P. Dudnik, "The Medical Effect of Magnetic-laser Therapy in Patients with Diabetic Angiopathies of the Lower Extremities," *Lik Sprava,* (10–12), October-December 1996, pp. 155–158.

R.A. Kuliev & R.F. Babaev, "A Magnetic Field in the Combined Treatment of Suppurative Wounds in Diabetes Mellitus," *Vestn Khir Im I I Grek,* 148(1), January 1992, pp. 33–36.

This study involving 72 diabetics with purulent wounds found that magnetic fields aided healing significantly.

R.A. Kuliev, et al., "Treatment of Suppurative Wounds in Patients with Diabetes Mellitus Magnetic Field and Laser Irradiation," *Khirurgliia,* (7-8), 1992, pp. 30–33.

V.A. Lebedev, "Treatment of Neurogenic Dysfunction of the Bladder and Enuresis in Children with a SKENAR Apparatus," *Vopr Kurortol Fizioter Lech Fiz Kult,* (4), 1995, pp. 25–26.

L.G. Vassilenko, "EHF Electromagnetic Radiation in Treatment of Obliterating Diseases of Inferior Limb Vessels," Second World Congress for Electricity and Magnetism in Biology and Medicine, 8–13 June 1997, Bologna, Italy.

DISEASES OF THE LARYNX

D.I. Tarasov, et al., "Effectiveness of Local Magnetic Field of the Acoustic Frequency in the Treatment of Patients with Acute Inflammatory Diseases of the Larynx," *Vestn Otorinolaringol,* (6), November-December 1995, pp. 11–15.

Results of this study found that alternative magnetic field of sound frequency proved to be an effective treatment in patients suffering from acute inflammatory diseases of the larynx.

DUCHENNE-ERB DISEASE

A.D. Burigina, et al., "Electromagnetic Waves in Complex Therapy of Children with Birth Trauma: Effects of Ultra-High-Frequency Electric Fields on Central Hemodynamics and the Shoulder Plexus," *Vopr Kurortol Fizioter Lech Fiz Kult,* (4), 1992, 35–38.

This study examined the effects of electromagnetic fields in the treatment of 5-year-old children suffering from Duchenne-Erb disease. Children were exposed to either UHF or DMW therapy for 8–12 minutes per day on alternating days over a period of approximately 10 days. Following the electromagnetic fields course, children received mud applications on the collar area and injured extremity. Results showed that treatment decreased contractures in shoulder and elbow joints, increased mobility and muscle strength, and improved general function of the arm.

ENDOMETRIOSIS

M. Damirov, et al., "Magnetic-Infrared-Laser Therapeutic Apparatus (MILTA) in Treatment of Patients with Endometriosis," *Vrach*, 12, 1994, pp. 17–19.

This study found that a combined treatment consisting of magnetic-infrared-laser therapy (10-15 min/day every other day over a period of 10–14 exposures, then repeated in 2–3 months) and conventional drug therapy proved highly effective in women suffering from endometriosis.

ENDOMETRITIS

V.M. Strugatskii, et al., "A Permanent Magnetic Field in the Combined Treatment of Acute Endometritis After an Artificial Abortion," *Vopr Kurortol Fizioter Lech Fiz Kult*, (6), November–December 1996, pp. 21–24.

Results of this study found that the administration of constant magnetic field in combination with other treatment modalities led to significant beneficial effects in patients suffering from acute endometritis following abortion.

EPILEPSY

P.A. Anninos, et al., "Magnetic Stimulation in the Treatment of Partial Seizures," *International Journal of Neurosci,* 60(3–4), October 1991, pp. 141–171.

This article reports on the cases of three patients with partial seizures who received treatment with external artificial magnetic fields of low intensity. Such treatment led to a significant attenuation of seizure frequency over a 10–14-month period.

G.D. Antimonii & R.A. Salamov, "Action of a Modulated Electromagnetic Field on Experimentally Induced Epileptiform Brain Activity in Rats," *Biull Eksp Biol Med,* 89(2), February 1980, pp. 145–148.

Experimental results indicated that the administration of modulated electromagnetic fields of 2–30 Hz suppressed epilepsy in rats.

M.J. McLean, et al., "Therapeutic Efficacy of a Static Magnetic Device in Three Animal Seizure Models: Summary of Experience," Second World Congress for Electricity and Magnetism in Biology and Medicine, 8–13 June 1997, Bologna, Italy.

This review article cites one study in particular in which results showed that pretreatment with 30 minutes of exposure to a 75-mT pole strength, DC-powered magnetic field significantly prevented experimentally induced seizures in mice.

F. Sartucci, et al., "Human Exposure to Oscillating Magnetic Fields Produces Changes in Pain Perception and Pain-Related Somatosensory Evoked Potentials," Second World Congress for Electricity and Magnetism in Biology and Medicine, 8–13 June 1997, Bologna, Italy.

This double-blind, placebo-controlled study examined the effects of 2-hour exposure to weak magnetic fields (0.2–0.7 G, irregularly oscillating 0.026–0.067 Hz) produced 3 pairs of orthogonal Helmholtz coils on pain perception in healthy subjects. Results showed that magnetic treatment significantly reduced the perception of pain.

R. Sandyk & P.A. Anninos, "Attenuation of Epilepsy with Application of External Magnetic Fields: A Case Report," *International Journal of Neurosci,* 66(1-2), September 1992, pp. 75–85.

This article reports on the case of a severe epileptic who experienced a significant lessening of behavior disturbances and seizure frequency following treatment with low-frequency, external artificial magnetic fields.

R. Sandyk & P.A. Anninos, "Magnetic Fields Alter the Circadian Periodicity of Seizures," *International Journal of Neurosci,* 63 (3–4), April 1992, pp. 265–274.

Low-frequency, external artificial magnetic field treatment was shown to significantly reduce seizures in four adult epileptic cases.

Gastroduodenitis

V.I. Bulynin, et al., "The Restoration of Esophageal Patency in Cicatricial Strictures Using Magnetic Elements," *Grud Serdechnososudistaia Khir*, (3), May–June 1993, pp. 53–56.

E.A. Luzhnikov, et al., "The Use of Magnetic Hemotherapy in Combined Detoxification in Acute Exogenous Poisonings," *Klin Med*, 73(3), 1995, pp. 37–40.

L.M. Petrukhina, et al., "Effect of a Decimeter Wave Electromagnetic Fields on the Motor Function of the Stomach in Children with Strong Gastroduodenitis," *Vopr Kurortol Fizioter Lech Fiz Kult*, (1), 1987, pp. 54–56.

Results of this study indicated that treatment with decimeter-band electromagnetic fields improved motor function of the stomach and reduced dyspepsia and pain in children suffering from chronic gastroduodenitis. Treatment made use of the "Romashka" apparatus (a cylinder applicator, 100 mm in diameter, power of 6–8 W) applied to the gastroduodenal region, and consisted of 6–12 minute exposures every other day for a total of 8–12 exposures.

O.V. Bukanovich, et al., "Sinusoidally-Modulated Currents in the Therapy of Chronic Gastroduodenitis in Children," *Vopr Kurortol Fizioter Lech Fiz Kult*, 2, 1996, pp. 22–26.

This controlled study examined the effects of sinusoidally modulated currents (100 Hz) coupled with conventional therapy in children suffering from chronic gastroduodenitis. Children received 8–10 exposures lasting between 6 and 10 minutes. Results showed that the treatment reduced inflammation in 72 percent of patients relative to just a 45 percent rate among controls. About 77 percent of treatment patients experienced elimination of gastro esophageal and duodeno-gastral refluxes, compared to 29 percent of controls.

GENERAL

L. Navratil, et al., "Possible Therapeutic Applications of Pulsed Magnetic Fields," *Cas Lek Cesk,* 132(19), October 11, 1993, pp. 590–594.

Results of this study indicated that the optimal frequency of pulsed magnetic fields ranges between 10.0 and 25.0 Hz in the treatment of chronic inflammatory conditions of the locomotor apparatus, ischemia of the blood vessels of the lower extremities, dyspeptic syndrome, lactation mastitis, and other diseases. Treatment proved best when the therapeutic cycle was repeated after a 2–3 month period.

J. Jerabek, "Pulsed Magnetotherapy in Czechoslovakia—A Review," *Rev Environ Health,* 10(2), April–June 1994, pp. 127–134.

This article reviews the use of magnetotherapy in Czechoslovakia. Noting that this modality has been used for more than a decade, the author states that magnetotherapy has been shown to be effective in treating rheumatic diseases, sinusitis, enuresis, and ischemic disorders of the lower extremities. Positive findings have also been shown with respect to multiple sclerosis and degenerative diseases of the retina.

A.A. Pilla, "State of the Art in Electromagnetic Therapeutics: Soft Tissue Applications," Second World Congress for Electricity and Magnetism in Biology and Medicine, 8–13 June 1997, Bologna, Italy.

This review article notes that pulse-type electromagnetic fields (PEMF) are the most frequently used type of electromagnetic therapy. Another form is pulsed radio frequency; PRF therapy generally includes daily sessions of 30-minute exposure and is primarily used in cases of pain and edema, with results being apparent quickly when the therapy is effective. PEMF treatment is most successful when used in bone healing, with results occurring over a longer period of time.

G. Annaratone, et al., "Magnetotherapy in Clinical and Ambulatory Practice," *Minerva Med*, 74(14–15), April 7, 1983, pp. 823–833.

This study examined the effects of electromagnetic fields administered over a period of 10 days on 354 patients suffering from various orthopedic conditions. Results showed the effects to be positive, with the greatest benefit experienced among patients with acute lesions.

C.A. Bassett, "Fundamental and Practical Aspects of Therapeutic Uses of Pulsed Electromagnetic Fields (PEMFs)," *Crit Rev Biomed Eng*, 17(5), 1989, pp. 451–529.

Noting that beneficial effects of low-energy, time-varying magnetic fields have been shown since the early 1970s, this review article cites studies pointing to its success in the treatment of a wide range of conditions. The best results for this modality obtained in the area of bone healing.

C.A. Bassett, "Beneficial Effects of Electromagnetic Fields," *Journal of Cell Biochem,* 51(4), April 1993, pp. 387–393.

This review article claims that over a quarter of a million patients worldwide with chronically ununited fractures have experienced beneficial results from treatment with pulsed electromagnetic fields. In addition, the author cites studies pointing to the treatment's efficacy with respect to other conditions such as nerve regeneration, wound healing, graft behavior, diabetes, heart attack, and stroke.

A.G. Pakhomov, "Millimeter Wave Medicine in Russia: A Review of Literature," Infrared Lasers and Millimeter Waves Workshop: The Links Between Microwaves and Laser Optics, January 21–22, 1997, Brooks Air Force Base, Texas.

This review article notes that low-intensity millimeter waves have been used for treating a wide variety of medical conditions in the former Soviet Union since 1977, with more than a million patients treated and more than a thousand treatment centers in existence. This therapy has been approved for widespread use by the Russian Ministry of Health, and over 300 scientific publications have described its effects. A typical course of treatment involves 10–15 daily exposures ranging from 15 to 60 minutes each.

S.D. Schvchenko, et al., "Experience with Treating Some Orthopedic Diseases with Millimeter Range Radiation of Nonthermal Intensity," *Millimeter Waves in Medicine and Biology.* Digest of Papers of the 11th Russian Symposium with International Participation, April 21–24, 1997, Zvenigorod, Moscow Region, Russia, pp. 33–35.

This study concluded that the use of millimeter wave (MW) therapy was effective in the treatment of both children and adults suffering from a variety of orthopedic diseases, including osteochondrosis, arthrosis, infantile cerebral paralysis, Perthes' disease, and inborn femur dislocation. MW therapy made use of the G4-142 apparatus (55–65 GHz). Exposure was for 15–30 minutes in children or 30–60 minutes in adults over a period of 10–12 total exposures.

A.M. Begue-Simon & R.A. Drolet, "Clinical Assessment of the Rhumart System based on the Use of Pulsed Electromagnetic Fields with Low Frequency," *International Journal of Rehabil Research,* 16(4), 1993, pp. 323–327.

This research examined the effects of low-frequency pulsed electromagnetic fields on patients suffering from a wide range of disorders, including musculoskeletal disorders, neurological disorders, circulatory diseases, traumatic disorders, gastroenterological problems, and stress-related morbidity. Treatment made use of the Rhumart apparatus, which produced waveforms with peak amplitudes up to 30 G. Results, based on the patients' own subjective ratings, indicated the treatment to be beneficial across most conditions, with the strongest effects seen in those suffering from musculoskeletal and traumatic disorders.

Y.L. Arzumanov, "An Overview of the Third Workshop 'Use of Millimeter Waves in Medicine,' " *Millimetrovie Volni v Biologii i Meditcine,* (3), 1994, pp. 104–107.

This review article summarizes findings presented at the Third Workshop on the use of low-intensity millimeter waves in medicine, held in Zvenigorod, Moscow Region, Russia. Such findings pointed to the efficacy of MW therapy with respect to alcoholism and its associated symptoms, gastric and duodenal ulcers, psoriasis, chronic furunculosis, and cardiovascular diseases.

N. Gilinskaya & L.V. Zobina, "Magnetic Field Application for the Treatment of Vascular Diseases of the Brain and Eyes," in Y.A. Kholodov & N.N. Lebedeva (eds.), *Problems of Electromagnetic Neurobiology,* Moscow, Nauka, 1988, pp. 94–98.

This study examined the effects of magnetotherapy on patients suffering from a variety of eye and brain vascular disorders. Treatment made use of the "Polius-1" apparatus (50 Hz), with most patients receiving a course of 15–20 daily exposures. Results showed overall general improvements in 95 percent of patients with eye diseases.

R.A. Drolet, "Rhumart Therapy: A Non-invasive Cell Regeneration Ion and Anti-Inflammatory Therapy Using LF-EM Fields," Bioelectromagnetics Society, 4th Annual Meeting, 28 June–2 July 1982, Los Angeles, CA, p. 45.

This review article notes that low-frequency electromagnetic therapy has been used for a variety of purposes. Those specifically identified by the author include cell growth promotion, pain reduction, improved blood circulation, bone repair, increased wound healing, sedative effects, enhanced sleep, and arthritic relief.

A. Zaslavskii, et al., "A Low-frequency Impulse Apparatus for Physical Therapy 'Infita'," *Med Tehk*, 5, 1994, pp. 39–41.

This review article notes that treatment with an "Infita" apparatus, used to deliver low-frequency magnetic fields, has been shown to improve general hemodynamics and microcirculation in addition to exhibiting anti-inflammatory, sedative, and analgesic effects in Olympic-level Russian athletes.

V.M. Bogoliubov & L.A. Skurikhina, "Therapeutic Application of Constant and Low-Frequency Magnetic Fields," *Vopr Kurortol Fizioter Lech Fiz Kult*, (2), 1979, pp. 65–72.

This review article cites studies pointing to the efficacy of low-frequency magnetic fields in the treatment of a wide variety of conditions, including burns, arthritis, fractures, arterial aneurysms, PMS, phantom pain, tuberculosis, ischemic heart disease, hypertension, bronchial asthma, and ulcerated varicose veins, among others.

V.I. Kovalchuk, et al., "Use of Extremely Low Frequency Magnetic Fields in Clinical Practice," *Fizicheskaia Meditzina*, 4(1–2), 1994, p. 87.

This study examined the effects of extremely-low-frequency magnetic fields (TAMMAT device) in the treatment of a group of 650 patients suffering from a host of various diseases. Treatment consisted of 15–25 minute daily exposures 5 days per week over a total of 20–25 days. Most patients experienced improvements after 2–3 exposures. Marked improvements were seen with respect to analgesic, anti-inflammatory, anti-tumor, and immune-enhancing effects.

S.A. Schastnyi, et al., "A Contact-Free, Biologically Adequate Electromagnetic Stimulation of Repair Regeneration of Osseous, Cartilaginous, and Muscular Tissues in Children," *Vestn Ross Akad Med Nauk,* (3), 1994, pp. 38–42.

This article reports on the efficacy of a Russian electromagnetic stimulation apparatus termed "Cascade." The authors state that data from 508 patients suffering from various ailments who were treated with the device indicate it to be anywhere from 75 to 100 percent effective. Examples of conditions in which the device was used include stubborn fractures, posttraumatic contractures, crush syndrome, and Perthes' disease.

J. Jerabek, "Pulsed Magnetotherapy in Czechoslovakia: A Review," First World Congress for Electricity and Magnetism in Biology and Medicine, 14–19 June 1992, Lake Buena Vista, FL, p. 81.

This review article on the use of pulsed magnetotherapy in Czechoslovakia points to its efficacy across a variety of conditions, including joint problems, enuresis, multiple sclerosis, diabetes, and carpal tunnel syndrome.

N.M. Suvorova, "Treatment of Chronic Inflammatory Diseases of the Female Genitals Permanent Magnetic Field," *Akush Ginekol,* (9), 1977, pp. 62–63.

GLAUCOMA

Bisvas, et al., "Possibilities of Magnetotherapy in Stabilization of Visual Function in Patients with Glaucoma," *Vestn Oftalmol,* 112(1), January–March 1996, pp. 6–8.

In this study, patients with primary open-angle glaucoma with compensated intraocular pressure were administered magnetotherapy using an ATOS device with 33-mT magnetic field induction. The procedure was administered to a patient in a sitting posture with a magnetic inductor held before the eye. Sessions lasted 10 minutes and each course included 10 sessions. Following 4–5 months of therapy, results showed improved vision acuity of 0.16 diopters, on an average of 29 out of 30 eyes with vision acuity below 1.0.

V.D. Grigor'eva & N.E. Fedorova, "New Methodological Aspects in the Use of Cryotherapy, Ultrasound, Magnetotherapy and Therapeutic Physical Exercise in the Rehabilitation of Gonarthrosis Patients," *Vopr Kurortol Fizioter Lech Fiz Kult,* (2), March-April 1996, pp. 26–28.

HAIR LOSS

W.S. Maddin, et al., "The Biological Effects of a Pulsed Electrostatic with Specific Reference to Hair: Electrotrichogenesis," *International Journal of Dermatology,* 29(6), 1990, pp. 446–450.

This double-blind, placebo-controlled study examined the effects of pulsed electromagnetic fields on hair loss in men suffering from male pattern baldness. PEMF exposures were administered to the head for 12 minutes and were given weekly or twice weekly over a period of 36 weeks. Results found the PEMF treatment both prevented hair loss and promoted regrowth without side effects.

HEADACHE

O. Grunner, et al., "Cerebral Use of a Pulsating Magnetic Field in Neuropsychiatry Patients with Long-term Headache," *EEG EMG Z Elektroenzephalogr Verwandte Geb,* 16(4), December 1985, pp. 227–230.

Results of this double-blind, placebo-controlled study demonstrated that the administration of a pulsed magnetic field for less than one hour to headache patients produced significant beneficial effects, as shown by subjective patient reports, as well as EEG activity.

R. Sandyk, "The Influence of the Pineal Gland on Migraine and Cluster Headaches and Effects of Treatment with picoTesla Magnetic Fields," *International Journal of Neurosci,* 67(1–4), November–December 1992, pp. 145–171.

This article reports on the case of an acute migraine patient who was successfully treated with external magnetic fields.

B.M. Popov & T.A. Al'shanskaya, "Use of Traditional and Non-traditional Methods in the Treatment of Headache," *Millimeter Waves in Medicine and Biology*. Digest of Papers of the 11th Russian Symposium with International Participation, April 21–24, 1997, Zvenigorod, Moscow Region, Russia, pp. 68–71.

This article examined the effects of millimeter wave therapy in the treatment of 107 patients suffering from headaches of varying causes. Treatment consisted of the Nao-Hu, Bai-Huei, and Hua-Chai acupuncture points being exposed to 5.6- and 4.9-mm wavelengths via the use of "Yav'-1-5.6" or "Electronka-KVCh" devices, respectively. Exposure lasted up to 60 minutes per day over a course of 10 days. All patients experienced positive results following 3–5 exposures. After one year, 48 percent of patients remained free of headaches, with a significant decrease in another 41 percent.

A. Prusinski, et al., "Pulsating Electromagnetic Field in the Therapy of Headache," Hungarian Symposium on Magnetotherapy, 2nd Symposium, May 16–17, 1987, Szekesfehervar, Hungary, pp. 163–166.

This study examined the effects of pulsed electromagnetic fields (20 minutes per day for 15 days) in the treatment of patients suffering from chronic headaches. Results indicated the treatment to be most effective in patients suffering from tension headaches, with 88 percent of such patients reporting positive results. Beneficial results were also experienced by patients suffering from migraines (60 percent), cervical migraines (68 percent), and psychogenic headaches (60 percent).

A. Prusinksi, et al., "Pulsating Electromagnetic Field in the Therapy of Headache," *Journal of Bioelectr.*, 7(1), 1988, pp. 127–128.

In this study, 90 headache patients were treated with pulsating electromagnetic fields via large coils to the body for 20 minutes per day for a total of 15 days. Results found the treatment to be either excellent or good for those patients suffering from migraine, tension, and/or cervical headaches. Patients experiencing posttraumatic or cluster headaches did not experience such benefits.

J. Giczi & A. Guseo, "Treatment of Headache Pulsating Electromagnetic Field, a Preliminary Report," Hungarian Symposium on Magnetotherapy, 2nd Symposium, May 16–17, 1987, Szekesfehervar, Hungary, pp. 74–76.

Results of this study indicated that pulsating electromagnetic fields (12 Hz and 5 mT) were an effective prophylactic treatment for patients suffering from cervical and migraine headaches.

L. Lazar & A. Farago, "Experiences of Patients Suffering from Migraine-Type Headache Treated with Magnetotherapy," Hungarian Symposium on Magnetotherapy, 2nd Symposium, May 16-17, 1987, Szekesfehervar, Hungary, pp. 137–140.

This placebo-controlled, double-blind study examined the effects of pulsed electromagnetic fields (2–5 Hz and flux densities of 3–4 mT) on patients suffering from migraine headaches. PEMFs were administered to the head for 10–

15 minutes per day over a period of 30 days. Results showed a mean improvement level of 66 percent in patients receiving the treatment, compared to just 23 percent among controls.

HEMOPHILIA

V.V. Aleschenko & I.O. Pisanko, "EHF-Therapy for Hemophylic Arthropathy and Hemarthroses of the Knee Joint," *Millimeter Waves in Medicine and Biology.* Digest of Papers of the 10th Russian Symposium with International Participation, April 24–26, Moscow, Russia, 1995, pp. 61–63.

In this study, hemophiliacs suffering from joint hemorrhage received millimeter wave (MW) therapy at biologically active points beginning on the first day of hospital release. Adults were treated with an "Electronica-KVCh" device (61 GHz, 5 mW maximum power) and children were treated with a "Porog" device, which generates low-intensity wide-band MMW noise. Exposures in both groups lasted for 20–25 minutes per day and were extended over a period of 10 days. Results indicated the treatment to be more effective than conventional therapy with respect to alleviation of pain, need for medication, and other parameters.

HEPATITIS

A.A. Shul'diakov, et al., "Electromagnetic Radiation of Millimeter Range in Treatment of Children with Acute Viral Hepatitis," *Millimeter Waves in Medicine and Biology,* 10th

Russian Symposium with International Participation, April 24–26, 1995, Moscow, Russia, pp. 21–23.

This double-blind, placebo-controlled study examined the effects of millimeter wave therapy combined with conventional methods in the treatment of viral hepatitis in children. Making use of a "Yav'-1-5,6" or "Yav'-1-7,7" device, MW therapy involved 14–15 exposures of, on average, 30 minutes per day at wavelengths of either 5.6 or 7.1 mm. Results indicated the combined treatment to be more effective than conventional treatment only, leading to a more rapid restoration of liver function.

I.A. Il'inskii, et al., "Experience with the Use of Glucocorticosteroids and Magnetic Fields in the Intensive Therapy of Severe Forms of Viral Hepatitis," *Soviet Medicine*, 9, 1978, pp. 72–74.

Results of this study showed that the use of magnetic fields was effective in treating patients suffering from viral hepatitis who had previously not benefited from conventional drug therapies.

V.V. Krasnov & A.I. Shilenok, "Magnetotherapy of Hepatitis A and B in Children," *Pediatriia*, 10, 1991, pp. 54–57.

This study examined the effects of magnetotherapy in children suffering from various forms of viral hepatitis. Magnetotherapy consisted of alternating magnetic fields applied to the liver area daily over a total of 10–15 days. Results indicated magnetotherapy led to more rapid and trouble-free recovery.

HERNIATED DISK

K. Perjes, et al., "Effect of Magnetotherapy on Recovery After Herniated Disk Surgery," Hungarian Symposium on Magnetotherapy, 2nd Symposium, May 16–17, 1987, Szekesfehervar, Hungary, pp. 159–162.

This double-blind, placebo-controlled study examined the effects of magnetotherapy in patients following herniated disk surgery. Results showed that 52 percent of patients receiving the treatment compared to 30 percent of controls reported being free of symptoms at the time of hospital release.

HIP PROBLEMS

G. Gualtieri, et al., "The Effect Pulsed Electromagnetic Field Stimulation on Patients Treated of Hip Revesions with Trans-Femoral Approach," Second World Congress for Electricity and Magnetism in Biology and Medicine, 8–13 June 1997, Bologna, Italy.

This double-blind study examined the effects of pulsed electromagnetic fields on loosened hip prostheses. Results showed an increase of bone density in all patients receiving PEMF treatment compared to only 60 percent of controls. The authors argue such findings suggest PEMF elicits early bone reconstruction, which enhances early weight bearing.

K. Konrad, "Therapy with Pulsed Electromagnetic Fields in Aseptic Loosening of Total Hip Protheses: A Prospective Study," *Clinical Rheumatology*, 15(4), 1996, pp. 325–328.

This study examined the effects of pulsed electromagnetic fields (50 Hz, 50 G) in treating aseptic loosening of total hip prostheses. PEMF therapy consisted of 20 minutes per day for 6 days per week over a total of 20 such sessions and was begun, on average, a year and a half following the start of loosening. Results showed PEMF to have some beneficial effects with respect to loosened hip arthroplasties, although it was not effective in patients suffering severe pain due to extreme loosening.

A. Zaslavskii, et al., " 'ELEMAGS' Apparatus and Clinical Experience with its Use for Treatment of Hypoacusis and Otalgia in Children," *Med Tekh*, (2), 1995, pp. 40–41.

E.A. Stepanov, et al., "The Treatment of Intestinal Fistulae in Children by Applying a By-pass Anastomosis Using Magnetic Devices," *Khirurgiia*, (11-12), November–December 1992, pp. 93–95.

JOINT DISEASE

E. Riva Sanseverino, et al., "Therapeutic Effects of Pulsed Magnetic Fields on Joint Diseases," *Panminerva Med*, 34(4), October-December 1992, pp. 187–196.

Results of this 11-year study involving 3014 patients found pulsed magnetic field treatment at low frequencies and intensities to be a highly effective, side-effect-free therapy for joint disease.

KIDNEY PROBLEMS

V.E. Rodoman, et al., "The Effect of Magnetic and Laser Therapy on the Course of an Experimental Inflammatory Process in the Kidneys," *Urol Nefrol* (Mosk), (2), March–April 1993, pp. 17–20.

A.A. Li, et al., "The Use of an Impulse Magnetic Field in the Combined Therapy of Patients with Stone Fragments in the Upper Urinary Tract," *Vopr Kurortol Fizioter Lech Fiz Kult,* (3), May–June 1994, pp. 22–24.

V.A. Kiyatkin, "Pulsed Magnetic Field in Therapy of Patients with Secondary Chronic Pyelonephritis," Second World Congress for Electricity and Magnetism in Biology and Medicine, 8–13 June 1997, Bologna, Italy.

This review article notes that placebo-controlled studies have shown positive results concerning the use of pulsed magnetic field therapy in the treatment of secondary chronic pyelonephritis.

L.U. Bigliani, "The Use of Pulsing Electromagnetic Fields to Achieve Arthrodesis of the Knee Following Failed Total Knee Arthroplasty. A Preliminary Report," *Journal of Bone Joint Surg,* 65(4), April 1983, pp. 480–485.

L.D. Dorogaia & G.F. Uchaikin, "Use of Microwave Resonance Therapy in Complex Treatment of Laryngotracheitis in Children," Pediatriia, (1), 1995, p. 55–57.

A.E. Kucherenko & V.I. Shevchuk, "Treatment of Diseases of Limb Stumps with Alternating Current Magnetic Field," *Klin Khir*, 7, 47–49.

G. Laszlo & T. Tanay, "Comparative Evaluation of Magnetotherapy Treatment in Patients Suffering from Locomotor Disease," Hungarian Symposium on Magnetotherapy, 2nd Symposium, 16–17 May 1987, Szekesfehervar, Hungary, pp. 128–136.

I.M. Garber, "A Combined Method for Treating the Neurological Manifestations of Lumbar Osteochondrosis with a Low-Frequency Magnetic Field and the Vacuum Phonophoresis of Hydrocortisone and Trilon B," *Vopr Kurortol Fizioter Lech Fiz Kult*, (2), 1990, pp. 61–62.

LUNG DISEASE

L.V. Iashchenko, "Low-Frequency Magnetic Fields in the Combined Therapy of Inflammatory Lung Diseases," *Probl Tuberk*, 3, 1988, pp. 53–56.

This study examined the effects of low-frequency magnetic fields coupled with conventional therapies in rats suffering from inflammatory lung disease. Results showed that rats receiving the magnetic fields experienced significant reductions in lung abscesses and associated symptoms, and similar beneficial effects were seen among a group of 165 human patients receiving comparable treatment.

Lupus Erythematosus

I.V. Khamaganova, et al., "The Use of a Pulsed Magnetic Field in the Treatment of Lupus Erythematosus," *Ter Arkh*, 67(10), 1995, pp. 84–87.

This review article examined the data concerning impulsed magnetic fields in the treatment of lupus erythematosus. Studies indicate that the treatment can be beneficial due to its anti-inflammatory and analgesic effects, its positive action on microcirculation, and immunological reactivity.

V.D. Sidorov & S.B. Pershin, "Immunomodulating Effect of Microwaves and Ultrahigh Frequency Electric Fields in Patients with Systemic Lupus Erythmatosus," *Bioelectrochem Bioenerg*, 30, 1993, pp. 327–330.

This double-blind, placebo-controlled study examined the effects of UHF and microwave therapy in treating patients suffering from systemic lupus. Twenty-six patients were given 30–35 W of microwave irradiation administered to the adrenal region. Twenty-five patients were given 30–35 W UHF administered bilaterally to the temporal region. The treatment regimen for both groups included 18–20 daily sessions. A group of 11 patients were used as controls. Results showed both treatments to be effective, with 27 percent of microwave patients and 66 percent of UHF patients reporting total elimination of polyarthralgia, myalgia, and painful contractures.

V.D. Sidorov, "The Immunomodulating Effect of Micro-waves and of an Ultrahigh Frequency Electrical Field in Patients with Systemic Lupus Erythematosus," *Vopr Kurortol Fizioter Lech Fiz Kult,* (4), 1991, pp. 36-40.

M.P. Nikolaev, et al., "The Clinico-immunological Assessment of the Efficacy of Magnetic-laser Therapy in Patients with Chronic Maxillary Sinusitis," *Vestn Otorinolaringol,* (2), March–April 1994, pp. 27-31.

Results of this study indicated that the bitemporal application of ultrahigh-frequency electromagnetic fields to the hypothalamo-hypophyseal area daily over a period of 18-20 days had beneficial effects in patients suffering from systemic lupus erythematosus.

Multiple Sclerosis

R. Sandyk, "Rapid Normalization of Visual Evoked Potentials picoTesla Range Magnetic Fields in Chronic Progressive Multiple Sclerosis," *International Journal of Neurosci,* 77(3–4), August 1994, pp. 243–259.

This article reports on the case of a 55-year-old female chronic progressive multiple sclerosis patient who received a single external application of low magnetic fields (7.5-picotesla; 5-Hz frequency) which lasted 20 minutes. The treatment quickly led to improvements in a variety of areas, including fatigue, sleep, vision, bladder function, movement and speech problems, and mood.

R. Sandyk, "Further Observations on the Effects of External picoTesla Range Magnetic Fields on Visual Memory and Visuospatial Functions in Multiple Sclerosis," *International Journal of Neurosci,* 77(3–4), August 1994, 203–27

This study reports on four cases of multiple sclerosis who experienced improvements in visuospatial and visuomotor functions following treatment with external application of low magnetic fields.

R. Sandyk, "Successful Treatment of Multiple Sclerosis with Magnetic Fields," *International Journal Neurosci,* 66(3–4), October 1992, pp. 237–250.

This article reports on the case of a 50-year-old female chronic progressive multiple sclerosis patient who received a single external application of low magnetic fields who experienced significant improvements following the treatment.

R. Sandyk, "Progressive Cognitive Improvement in Multiple Sclerosis from Treatment with Electromagnetic Fields," *International Journal of Neurosci,* 89(1–2), January 1997, pp. 39–51.

This article reports on the cases of three patients suffering from long-time symptoms of multiple sclerosis who received treatment with extracerebral pulsed electromagnetic fields over a period of between 6 and 18 months. Results showed all three patients experienced significant improvements in cognitive functions.

R. Sandyk, "Resolution of Dysarthria in Multiple Sclerosis Treatment with Weak Electromagnetic Fields," *International Journal of Neurosci*, 83(1–2), November 1995, pp. 81–92.

This is a report on the cases of two chronic multiple sclerosis patients exhibiting severe speech problems. Symptoms were completely resolved following 3–4 weeks of treatment with pulsed electromagnetic fields.

R. Sandyk, "Reversal of Alexia in Multiple Sclerosis by Weak Electromagnetic Fields," *International Journal of Neurosci*, 83(1–2), November 1995, pp. 69–79.

This article reports on the cases of three multiple sclerosis patients suffering from alexia (lack of understanding of written words) who experienced a reversal of the alexia following the start of picotesla-range electromagnetic field treatment.

R. Sandyk, "Long Term Beneficial Effects of Weak Electromagnetic Fields in Multiple Sclerosis," *International Journal of Neurosci*, 83(1–2), November 1995, pp. 45–57.

This article reports on the case of a middle-aged disabled female patient with a 19-year history of chronic relapsing-remitting multiple sclerosis. Within one day of receiving experimental treatment with picotesla electromagnetic fields, the patient exhibited improvements in her condition. The patient continued with 1–2 treatments per week over a period of 32 months. During this time, significant improvements were seen with respect to a range of physical symptoms, as well as cognitive functions.

R. Sandyk, "Suicidal Behavior is Attenuated in Patients with Multiple Sclerosis Treatment with Electromagnetic Fields," *International Journal of Neurosci*, 87(1–2) October 1996, pp. 5–15.

The cases of three female multiple sclerosis patients exhibiting suicidal behavior are discussed in this article. Treatment with pulsed picotesla-level electromagnetic fields resolved the suicidal behavior in all three patients, an improvement that was maintained over a follow-up period of 3.5 years.

R. Sandyk, "Treatment with Electromagnetic Field Alters the Clinical Course of Chronic Progressive Multiple Sclerosis—A Case Report," *International Journal of Neurosci*, 88(1–2), November 1996, pp. 75–82.

This article reports on the case of a 36-year-old man severely disabled with partial paralysis and lack of coordination. Three treatment sessions per week with pulsed electromagnetic fields over a period of one year led to a range of improvements, including improvements in gait, balance, bowel and bladder functions, vision, mood, and slee pp. No progression of symptoms associated with multiple sclerosis was seen throughout the course of EMF treatment.

R. Sandyk, "Effect of Weak Electromagnetic Fields on Body Image Perception in Patients with Multiple Sclerosis," *International Journal of Neurosci*, 86(1–2), July 1996, pp. 79–85.

This article reports on the cases of two multiple sclerosis patients suffering from chronic ataxia who performed poorly on human figure drawing tests administered to measure body image perception. Treatment with extracerebral applications of picotesla flux electromagnetic fields led to improvements in gait and balance as well as a normalization in body image perception as seen on a repeat of the same test by each patient.

R. Sandyk, "Treatment with Weak Electromagnetic Fields Attenuates Carbohydrate Craving in a Patients with Multiple Sclerosis," *International Journal of Neurosci*, 86(1–2), July 1996, pp. 67–77.

This article reports on the case of a 51-year-old female patient with remitting-progressive multiple sclerosis who experienced a successful reduction in carbohydrate craving believed to be associated with the exacerbation of her condition following treatment with a series of extracranial AC pulsed applications of picotesla flux intensity by electromagnetic fields.

R. Sandyk, "Reversal of an Acute Parkinsonian Syndrome Associated with Multiple Sclerosis Application of Weak Electromagnetic Fields," *International Journal of Neurosci*, 86(1–2), July 1996, pp. 33–45.

R. Sandyk & L.C. Dann, "Resolution of Lhermitte's Sign in Multiple Sclerosis Treatment with Weak Electromagnetic Fields," *International Journal of Neurosci*, 81(3–4), April 1995, pp. 215–224.

R. Sandyk & L.C. Dann, "Weak Electromagnetic Fields Attenuate Tremor in Multiple Sclerosis," *International Journal of Neurosci*, 79(3–4), December 1994, pp. 199–212.

This article reports on the cases of three multiple sclerosis patients suffering from a chronic progressive course of the disease who experienced a reduction in tremors following treatment with brief external applications of pulsed EMFs of 7.5-pT intensity.

R. Sandyk, "Reversal of Visuospatial Hemi-inattention in Patients with Chronic Progressive Multiple Sclerosis by Treatment with Weak Electromagnetic Fields," *International Journal of Neurosci*, 79(3–4), December 1994, pp. 169–184.

This article reports on the cases of three female chronic multiple sclerosis patients who experienced a reversal of cognitive deficits following treatment with brief external applications of alternating pulsed electromagnetic fields in the picotesla range of intensity.

R. Sandyk, "Improvement in Word-fluency Performance in Patients with Multiple Sclerosis Electromagnetic Fields," *International Journal Neurosci*, 79(1–2), November 1994, pp. 75–90.

This article reports on the cases of three female multiple sclerosis patients with poor word fluency who experienced a 100-percent increase in word output following 4-5 sessions of treatment with external applications of extremely weak electromagnetic fields in the picotesla range of intensity.

R. Sandyk & R.P. Iacono, "Improvement PicoTesla Range Magnetic Fields of Perceptual-motor Performance and Visual Memory in a Patient with Chronic Progressive Multiple Sclerosis," *International Journal of Neurosci*, 78(1–2), September 1994, pp. 53–66.

This article reports on the case of a 58-year-old male multiple sclerosis patient with a 37-year history of the disease. Treatment with external application of magnetic fields in the picotesla range led to a speedy improvement of neurological symptoms in the areas of walking, balance, sensory symptoms, and bladder function. Improvements in numerous cognitive functions were seen within 24 hours of treatment as well.

R. Sandyk & R.P. Iacono, "Multiple Sclerosis: Improvement of Visuoperceptive Functions PicoTesla Range Magnetic Fields," *International Journal of Neurosci*, 74(1–4), January-February 1994, pp. 177–189.

This article reports on the case of a 36-year-old multiple sclerosis patient who experienced immediate improvements in visuoperceptive functions following treatment with external application of picotesla-range magnetic fields.

R. Sandyk, "Application of Weak Electromagnetic Fields Facilitates Sensory-motor Integration in Patients with Multiple Sclerosis," *International Journal of Neurosci*, 85(1–2), March 1996, pp. 101–110.

This article reports on the cases of three multiple sclerosis patients suffering from falls due to rapid deterioration in balance and triggered by distracting external auditory stimuli. Treatment with a series of extracranially applied, low-frequency picotesla-range intensity electromagnetic fields quickly resolved such symptoms associated with a loss of balance.

R. Sandyk, "Treatment with Weak Electromagnetic Fields Improves Fatigue Associated with Multiple Sclerosis," *International Journal of Neurosci*, 84(1–4), February 1996, pp. 177–186.

This article reports on the cases of three multiple sclerosis patients experiencing continuous and debilitating daily fatigue over the course of several years. Treatment with extracranially applied picotesla flux electromagnetic fields dramatically improved symptoms of fatigue in all three patients.

R. Sandyk, "Resolution of Partial Cataplexy in Multiple Sclerosis Treatment with Weak Electromagnetic Fields," *International Journal of Neurosci*, 84(1–4), February 1996, pp. 157–164.

R. Sandyk, "Weak Electromagnetic Fields Restore Dream Recall in Patients with Multiple Sclerosis," *International Journal of Neurosci*, 82(1–2), May 1995, pp. 113–125.

R. Sandyk, "Weak Electromagnetic Fields Improve Body Image Perception in Patients with Multiple Sclerosis," *International Journal of Neurosci*, 82(3–4), June 1995, pp. 285–302.

R. Sandyk, "Premenstrual Exacerbation of Symptoms in Multiple Sclerosis is Attenuated by Treatment with Weak Electromagnetic Fields," *International Journal of Neurosci*, 83(3–4), December 1995, pp. 187–198.

This article reports on the cases of two female patients with chronic progressive-stage multiple sclerosis who suffered from regular worsening of their symptoms starting approximately a week prior to menstruation and abating at menstruation onset. Such symptoms were resolved in both patients two months following the start of treatment with the extracranial application of weak electromagnetic fields.

R. Sandyk & K. Derpapas, "Successful Treatment of an Acute Exacerbation of Multiple Sclerosis by External Magnetic Fields," *International Journal of Neurosci*, 70(1–2), May 1993, pp. 97–105.

R. Sandyk & R.P. Iacono, "Resolution of Longstanding Symptoms of Multiple Sclerosis by Application of PicoTesla Range Magnetic Fields," *International Journal of Neurosci*, 70(3–4), June 1993, pp. 255–269.

This article reports on the case of a 64-year-old female patient with a 22-year history of chronic progressive multiple sclerosis. Two 30-minute treatments with low-level electromagnetic fields produced a marked improvement in a variety of symptoms.

R. Sandyk & K. Derpapas, "Magnetic Fields Normalize Visual Evoked Potentials and Brainstem Auditory Evoked Potentials in Multiple Sclerosis," *International Journal of Neurosci*, 68(3–4), February 1993, pp. 241–253.

A. Guseo, "Double-Blind Treatments with Pulsating Electromagnetic Field in Multiple Sclerosis," Hungarian Symposium on Magnetotherapy, 2nd Symposium, May 16–17, 1987, Szekesfehervar, Hungary, pp. 85–89.

Results of this double-blind, placebo-controlled study found that pulsed electromagnetic fields administered daily over a period of 15 days proved to be an effective treatment in reducing spasticity and incontinence associated with multiple sclerosis.

A. Guseo, "Pulsing Electromagnetic Field Therapy of Multiple Sclerosis the Gyuling-Bordacs Device: Double-Blind, Cross-Over and Open Studies," *Journal of Bioelectr*, 6(1), 1987, pp. 23–35.

Results of this double-blind, placebo-controlled study indicated that pulsed electromagnetic fields administered daily over a period of 15 days is a generally effective treatment in reducing symptoms associated with multiple sclerosis, with the most positive improvements involving the alleviation of spasticity and pain.

A. Sieron, et al., "The Variable Magnetic Fields in the Complex Treatment of Neurological Diseases," European Bioelectromagnetics Association, 3rd International Congress, 29 February–3 March 1996, Nancy, France.

Results of this double-blind, placebo-controlled study indicated that exposure to magnetic fields produced beneficial clinical effects in patients suffering from cerebral paralysis and in patients with multiple sclerosis.

MUSCLE INJURY

I.E. Detlav, "The Influence of Constant and Pulsed Electromagnetic Fields on Oxidation Processes in Muscle," in I.E. Detlav, (ed.), *Electromagnetic Therapy of Injuries and Diseases of the Support-Motor Apparatus.* International Collection of Papers, Riga, Latvia: Riga Medical Institute, 1987, pp. 12–16.

This study examined the effects of pulsed electromagnetic fields on recovery following muscle injury in rats. Results showed that both pulsed and constant magnetic fields were equally effective, with the constant field being more intense.

L. Mecseki, et al., "The Study of the Efficacy of Magnetotherapy in Peripheral Paralysis," Hungarian Symposium on Magnetotherapy, 2nd Symposium, 16–17 May 1987, Szekesfehervar, Hungary, pp. 149–158.

This study examined the effects of pulsed electromagnetic fields (Gyuling-Bordacs device) in patients suffering from peripheral muscle paralysis. Treatment consisted of 20-minute exposures (2–50 Hz, 70 G). Results showed 50-Hz pulsed electromagnetic fields to be the most effective level of treatment and that such therapy enhanced muscle irritability in peripheral paralysis patients as well as in healthy controls.

NECK PAIN

D. Foley-Nolan, et al., "Low Energy High Frequency (27.12 MHZ) Therapy for Persistent Neck Pain. Double Blind Placebo Controlled Trial," *Bioelectromagnetics Society*, 12th Annual, June 10–14, 1990, San Antonio, TX, pp. 73.

This double-blind, placebo-controlled study examined the effects of low-energy pulsed electromagnetic fields administered via soft collars on patients suffering from persistent neck pain. Results indicated significantly beneficial effects following three weeks of treatment.

NERVE DAMAGE

H. Ito & C.A. Bassett, "Effect of Weak, Pulsing Electromagnetic Fields on Neural Regeneration in the Rat," *Clin Orthop*, (181), December 1983, pp. 283–290.

This controlled study found that exposure to pulsed electromagnetic fields enhanced the speed and degree of peripheral nerve regeneration twofold in rats with experimentally severed sciatic nerves.

A.R. Raji & R.E. Bowden, "Effects of High-peak Pulsed Electromagnetic Field on the Degeneration and Regeneration of the Common Peroneal Nerve in Rats," *Journal of Bone Joint Surg,* 65(4), August 1983, pp. 478–492.

Results of this controlled study demonstrated that treatment with 15 minutes per day of pulsed electromagnetic fields enhanced recovery time of experimentally injured nerves in rats.

M.G. Orgel, et al., "Pulsing Electromagnetic Field Therapy in Nerve Regeneration: An Experimental Study in the Cat," *Plast Reconstr Surg,* 73(2), February 1984, pp. 173–183.

O.A. Krylov, et al., "The Action of an Impulse Magnetic Field on the Motor Function Recovery of the Peripheral Nerve Trunks," *Vopr Kurortol Fizioter Lech Fiz Kult,* (6), November-December 1991, pp. 40–44.

A.M. Raji, "An Experimental Study of the Effects of Pulsed Electromagnetic Field (Diapulse) on Nerve Repair," *Journal of Hand Surg,* 9(2), June 1984, pp. 105–112.

Results of this study indicated that the use of pulsed electromagnetic fields on experimentally divided and sutured nerves in rats sped up regeneration of damaged nerves and the time it took for limb use to be recovered.

L.V. Zobina, et al., "Effectiveness of Magnetotherapy in Optic Nerve Atrophy. A Preliminary Study," _Vestn Oftalmol,_ 106(5), September–October 1990, pp. 54–57.

This study examined the effects of a Soviet Polyus-1 low-frequency magnetotherapy device used to administer approximately 10 mT for approximately 10 minutes in patients with optic nerve atrophy. Patients underwent 10–15 sessions per course. Results showed that vision acuity in patients with low acuity values (below 0.04 diopters) improved in 50 percent of cases. It was also found that the treatment improved ocular blood flow in cases of optic nerve atrophy. Optimal benefits were experienced after 10 therapy sessions.

NEUROLOGICAL DISORDERS

G. Terlaki, "Clinical Experiences by Magnetotherapy," Hungarian Symposium on Magnetotherapy, 2nd Symposium, 16–17 May 1987, Szekesfehervar, Hungary, pp. 175–179.

This article summarizes clinical results obtained by the authors in using pulsed electromagnetic fields (Gyuling-Bordacs device) in the treatment of neurological and locomotor disorders among a group of 148 patients in a hospital setting over a period of 3 years. The authors claim that 58–80 percent of such patients experienced benefits of some kind over the course of magnetotherapy.

A.A. Skorometz, et al., "Magnetic Impulse Therapy of Patients with Spondylogenic Diseases of the Nervous System," _Fizicheskaia Meditzina,_ 3(1-2), 1993, pp. 41–43.

This study examined the effects of magnetotherapy on patients suffering from nervous system diseases. Treatment consisted of 10–12 6-minute exposures (10–20 kG, 0.1–0.6 Hz). Results indicated beneficial effects in 25 of the 27 patients receiving the treatment.

A.G. Shiman, et al., "Use of Combined Methods of Magnetoelectrotherapy in the Treatment for Polineuropathies," *Vopr Kurortol Fizioter Lech Fiz Kult*, (5), 1993, pp., 38–41.

Results of this study found that the use of magnetic fields (30–35 mT, 10 and 100 Hz) produced beneficial effects in 93 percent of patients suffering from nerve problems.

OSTEOARTHRITIS

D.H. Trock, et al., "The Effect of Pulsed Electromagnetic Fields in the Treatment of Osteoarthritis of the Knee and Cervical Spine. Report of Randomized, Double Blind, Placebo Controlled Trials," *Journal of Rheumatology*, 21(10), 1994, pp. 1903–1911.

Results of this double-blind, placebo-controlled study indicated that exposure to pulsed electromagnetic fields had beneficial effects in the treatment of patients suffering from painful osteoarthritis of the knee or cervical spine. PEMF therapy consisted of 18 exposures lasting 30 minutes and administered 3–5 times per week.

G. Markarov, et al., "Therapeutic Effectiveness of Infra-red Laser Ray Combined with Quasi-stationary Electromagnetic Field in Patients with Osteoarthrosis," Bioelectro-magnetics Society, 16th Annual Meeting, 12–17 June 1994, Copenhagen, Denmark, pp. 114–115.

D.H. Trock, et al., "Treatment of Osteoarthritis with Pulsed Electromagnetic Fields," Bioelectric Repair and Growth Society, Vol. XIII, 13th Annual Meeting, 10–13 October 1993, Dana Point, CA, pp. 14.

This double-blind, placebo-controlled study indicated that treatment with pulsed electromagnetic fields produced significant favorable effects in patients suffering from osteoarthritis.

A.J. Bollet, et al., "Treatment of Osteoarthritis with Pulsed Electromagnetic Fields," European Bioelectromagnetics Association, 2nd Congress, 9–11 December 1993, Bled Slovenia, pp. 46.

This double-blind, placebo-controlled study showed that treatment with pulsed electromagnetic fields yielded significant benefits in patients suffering from osteoarthritis of the knee or cervical spine. PEMF therapy (25 G, 5–24 Hz) consisted of 18 30-minute exposures over a period of 3–4 weeks.

L. Yurkiv, et al., "The Use of Changeable Magnetic Field in Treatment of Osteoarthrosis," European Bioelectromagnetics Association, 3rd International Congress, 29 February–3 March 1996, Nancy France.

This controlled study examined the effects of changeable magnetic fields (Polus-101 device) coupled with more conventional therapies in the treatment of patients suffering from osteoarthrosis. Magnetic therapy consisted of daily 20 minute exposures for a total of 12 sessions. Results showed more rapid improvements of immunological indices and alleviation of symptoms associated with the disease among patients receiving the combination therapy compared to those treated only conventionally.

OSTEOCHONDROSIS

L.L. Butenko, "The Use of Alternating Magnetic Fields in Spinal Osteochondrosis," *Mechanisms of Biological Action of Electromagnetic Fields*, 27–31 October 1987, Pushchino, USSR, USSR Academy of Sciences, Research Center for Biological Studies, Inst. of Biological Physics, Coordination Council of Comecon Countries and Yugoslavia for Research in the Fields of Biological Physics, pp. 183.

This study examined the effects of alternating magnetic fields (50 Hz, 10–50 mT) combined with conservative therapy in patients suffering from spinal osteochondrosis. Treatment consisted of 20-minute exposures over a total of 20–25 such exposures per course. Results showed clinical benefits in 95 percent of patients receiving the combination treatment compared to just 30 percent among controls.

OSTEONECROSIS

N.S. Eftekhar, et al., "Osteonecrosis of the Femoral Head Treated by Pulsed Electromagnetic Fields (PEMFs): A Preliminary Report," *Hip*, 1983, pp. 306–330.

This pilot study found that the use of pulsed electromagnetic fields produced beneficial effects in patients suffering from osteonecrosis of the femoral head.

M. Hinsenkamp, et al., "Preliminary Results in Electromagnetic Field Treatment of Osteonecrosis," *Bioelectrochem Bioenerg*, 30, 1993, pp. 229–236.

This study examined the use of pulsed electromagnetic fields in the treatment of osteonecrosis. Compared to published findings concerning surgical treatment, results showed PEMF therapy to be superior in producing improvement.

OSTEOPOROSIS

A. Zati, et al., "Effects of Pulsed Magnetic Fields in the Therapy of Osteoporosis Induced by Ovariectomy in the Rat," *Boll Soc Ital Biol Sper*, 69(7–8), July–August 1993, pp. 469–475.

This study examined the effects of pulsed electromagnetic fields on postmenopausal osteoporosis in 10-month-old female rats. Results showed that EMF treatment for one hour per day for 4 months with a 30-gauss maximum pulse reduced bone mass loss to within 10 percent, while a 70-gauss maximum pulse reduced bone mass loss entirely.

C.T. Rubin, et al., "Prevention of Osteoporosis by Pulsed Electromagnetic Fields," *Journal of Bone Joint Surg*, 71(3), March 1989, pp. 411–417.

S. Mishima, "The Effect of Long-term Pulsing Electromagnetic Field Stimulation on Experimental Osteoporosis of Rats," *Sangyo Ika Daigaku Zasshi*, 10(1), March 1, 1988, pp. 31–45.

This study examined the effects of long-term pulsing electromagnetic fields in the form of repetitive pulse burst waves over a period of 6 months in osteoporotic rats. Results showed increased bone volume and formation activity.

F. Tabrah, et al., "Bone Density Changes in Osteoporosis-prone Women Exposed to Pulsed Electromagnetic Fields (PEMFs)," *Journal of Bone Miner Res*, 5(5), May 1990, pp. 437–442.

This study examined the effects of a 72-Hz pulsating electromagnetic field administered for 10 hours per day over a period of 12 weeks on bone density in women prone to osteoporosis. Results found significant increases in bone mineral density in the area of EMF exposure.

T.W. Bilotta, et al., "The Use of Low-Frequency Low Magnitude PEMFs in Treatment of Osteoporosis," *Journal of Bioelectr*, 8(2), 1989, pp. 316.

In this study, osteoporosis patients received treatment with pulsed electromagnetic fields (50 G, 50–100 Hz) for 30 minutes per session over a period of two years involving 20 sessions. These subjects were compared to similar patients treated with calcitonin. Results indicated PEMF to be effective in reducing pain, and to be even more so when combined with the conventional drug treatment.

T.W. Bilotta, et al., "Influence of Pulsed Electromagnetic Fields on Post-Menopausal Osteoporosis," First World Congress for Electricity and Magnetism in Biology and Medicine, 14–19 June 1992, Lake Buena Vista, FL, pp. 78.

This controlled study examined the effects of pulsed electromagnetic fields in women suffering from postmenopausal osteoporosis. Treatment consisted of daily 30-minute exposures for 20 days every six months. Results showed that PEMF treatment combined with 100 IU per day of nasal spray synthetic salmon calcitonin arrested bone decrease and significantly increased bone mass relative to patients receiving drug therapy alone.

G. Saveriano & S. Ricci, "Treatment of Senile Osteoporosis Caused by Rachialgia with Low-Frequency PEMFs," *Journal of Bioelectr*, 8(2), 1989, pp. 321.

Results of this study found the use of total-body low-frequency magnetic fields (60 G, 50–100 Hz) to be effective in the treatment of patients suffering from osteoporosis-related symptoms. Treatment consisted of a total of 15 exposures of 30 minutes each.

OTITIS EXTERNA

V.V. Sunstov, "Treatment of Acute Diffuse Otitis Externa by Low-Frequency Magnetic Fields," *Vestn Otorinolaringol*, 6, 1991, pp. 35–38.

This study examined the effects of synchronizing pulse waves in the impaired area when treating patients suffering from acute diffuse otitis externa with low-level magnetic fields in combination with conventional therapies. Patients were divided into three groups. The first received ultra-high frequency or very high frequency electromagnetic waves. The second received 15-minute daily exposures to 50–Hz alternating or pulsating 20-mT magnetic fields. The third group of patients were treated by switching on the same magnetic fields only during propagation of the pulse wave through the ear vessels. Results showed a 100 percent recovery rate in patients across all three groups, with recovery taking the least amount of time among those in group 3.

PANCREATITIS

V.V. Kents, et al., "The Efficacy of the Combined Use of 5-fluorouracil Electrophoresis and Magnetotherapy in Experimental Pancreatitis," *Vopr Kurortol Fizioter Lech Fiz Kult*, (3), May–June 1994, pp. 17–19.

A.A. Fedorov, et al., "The Use of a Low-frequency Magnetic Field in the Combined Therapy of Chronic Pancreatitis," *Vopr Kurortol Fizioter Lech Fiz Kult*, (5), September–October 1990, pp. 28–30.

This study found that sinusoidal and continuous low-frequency alternating magnetic field generated by a Polius-1 apparatus exhibited beneficial effects in patients suffering from chronic pancreatitis.

O.G. Savina, et al., "A Low-Frequency Pulsed Current and a Low-Intensity Laser Radiation in the Treatment of Acute Pancreatitis," *Vopr Kurortol Fizioter Lech Fiz Kult*, (2), 1995, pp. 39–40.

This controlled study examined the effects of combining pulsed electric stimulation and laser light with conventional treatment in patients suffering from acute pancreatitis. Results showed the combined therapy to have the most significant effects in patients with severe forms of the disease.

PARKINSON'S DISEASE

R. Sandyk, "Brief Communication: Electromagnetic Fields Improve Visuospatial Performance and Reverse Agraphia in a Parkinsonian Patient," *International Journal of Neurosci*, 87(3–4), November 1996, pp. 209–217.

This article reports on the case of a 73-year-old male Parkinson's patient suffering from disabling resting and postural tremors in the right hand, as well as other symptoms. Two successive 20-minute treatments with AC pulsed electromagnetic fields of 7.5-picotesla intensity and 5-Hz frequency sinusoidal wave led to improvements in visuospatial performance and a legible signature. Significant improvements in Parkinsonian motor symptoms were also seen following additional treatments.

R. Sandyk & R.P. Iacono, "Reversal of Visual Neglect in Parkinson's Disease by Treatment with PicoTesla Range

Magnetic Fields," *International Journal of Neurosci*, 73(1–2), November 1993, pp. 93–107.

This article reports on the case of a medicated 61-year-old Parkinson's patient who experienced rapid reversal of symptoms following a single external application of picotesla-range magnetic fields.

R. Sandyk, "Magnetic Fields in the Therapy of Parkinsonism," *International Journal of Neurosci*, 66(3–4), October 1992, pp. 209–235.

This article reports on four Parkinson's patients who experienced significant improvement in symptoms following treatment with picotesla-range magnetic fields. Two additional patients suffering from Parkinson's-related dementia experienced significant improvements in visuospatial impairment.

M.S. George, et al., "Transcranial Magnetic Stimulation: A Neuropsychiatric Tool for the 21st Century," *Journal of Neuropsychiatry Clin Neurosci*, 8(4), Fall 1996, pp. 373–382.

Noting that transcranial magnetic stimulation (TMS) is a new and noninvasive method of direct cortical neuron stimulation, this review article discusses recent studies showing that TMS has led to improvements in symptoms associated with Parkinson's disease and depression.

J. Bardasano, et al., "Extracranial Device for Noninvasive Neurological Treatments with Pulsating ELF Magnetic Fields," Second World Congress for Electricity and Magnetism in Biology and Medicine, 8–13 June 1997, Bologna, Italy.

Results of this study showed that the application of ELF magnetic fields via a plastic helmet device housing a set of coils (generating fields of 8 Hz and 7.5 pT) produced beneficial clinical effects after 30 minutes in patients suffering Parkinson's disease and multiple sclerosis.

R. Sandyk, "Parkinsonian Micrographia Reversed by Treatment with Weak Electromagnetic Fields," *International Journal of Neurosci*, 81(1–2), March 1995, pp. 83–93.

This article reports on the cases of two Parkinson's patients who experienced improvements in motor symptoms following treatment with external application of weak electromagnetic fields in the picotesla range.

R. Sandyk, "Improvement in Short-term Visual Memory by Weak Electromagnetic Fields in Parkinson's Disease," *International Journal of Neurosci*, 81(1–2), March 1995, pp. 67–82.

This article reports on the cases of three Parkinson's patients on full medication who exhibited an improvement in right hemispheric functions following a series of treatments with external application of electromagnetic fields in the picotesla range.

R. Sandyk, "Weak Electromagnetic Fields Reverse Visuospatial Hemi-inattention in Parkinson's Disease," *International Journal of Neurosci*, 81(1–2), March 1995, pp. 47–65.

R. Sandyk, "A Drug Naive Parkinsonian Patient Successfully Treated with Weak Electromagnetic Fields," *International Journal of Neurosci*, 79(1–2), November 1994, pp. 99–110.

This article reports on the case of a nonmedicated 49-year-old male Parkinson's patient who experienced a dramatic improvement in motor, depressive, and cognitive symptoms following treatment with brief extracranial applications of picotesla-range electromagnetic fields.

R. Sandyk & R.P. Iacono, "Reversal of Micrographia in Parkinson's Disease Application of picoTesla Range Magnetic Fields," *International Journal of Neurosci* 77(1–2), July 1994, pp. 77–84.

This article reports on the case of a 61-year-old Parkinson's patient who experienced improvements in the severity of motor problems 30 minutes after treatment with external application of weak electromagnetic fields in the picotesla range. Sham treatment had no such effects in the same patient.

R. Sandyk, "Improvement in Word-fluency Performance in Parkinson's Disease by Administration of Electromagnetic Fields," *International Journal of Neurosci*, 77(1–2), July 1994, pp. 23–46.

This article reports on the cases of five Parkinsonian patients on full medication who experienced a marked improvement in performance on Thurstone's Word-Fluency Test following treatment with a series of extremely low intensity electromagnetic fields in the picotesla range and of 5–8 Hz frequency.

R. Sandyk, "Treatment of Parkinson's Disease with Magnetic Fields Reduces the Requirement for Antiparkinsonian Medications," *International Journal of Neurosci*, 74(1–4), January–February 1994, pp. 191–201.

This article reports on the case of a 69-year-old Parkinsonian patient who was able to discontinue most medication for two weeks following two treatment sessions with extracranial picotesla-range magnetic fields. Symptoms recurred after three weeks and the patient received four more magnetic field sessions on consecutive days after four weeks. The patient was then able to discontinue medications completely.

R. Sandyk, "Reversal of a Visuoconstructional Deficit in Parkinson's Disease Application of External Magnetic Fields: A Report of Five Cases," *International Journal of Neurosci*, 75(3–4), April 1994, pp. 213–228.

This article reports on the cases of five medicated Parkinsonian patients who experienced improvements in motor, behavioral, and autonomic functions, and in visuoconstructional tasks following treatment with extracranial application of magnetic fields in the picotesla range.

R. Sandyk, "Freezing of Gait in Parkinson's Disease is Improved by Treatment with Weak Electromagnetic Fields," *International Journal of Neurosci*, 85(1–2), March 1996, pp. 111–124.

This article reports on the cases of three medicated Parkinsonian patients who experienced relief from disabling periods of freezing gait following treatment with extracerebral applications of pulsed electromagnetic fields in the picotesla range.

R. Sandyk, "Improvement of Body Image Perception in Parkinson's Disease Treatment with Weak Electromagnetic Fields," *International Journal of Neurosci*, 82(3–4), June 1995, pp. 269–283.

The cases of four nondemented Parkinsonian patients under full medication are discussed in this article. These patients performed poorly on human figure drawing tests administered to measure body image perception. Treatment with extracerebral applications of picotesla-range intensity electromagnetic fields led to marked improvements in body image perception as seen on a repeat of the same test by each patient.

R. Sandyk, "Reversal of Visuospatial Deficit on the Clock Drawing Test in Parkinson's Disease by Treatment with Weak Electromagnetic Fields," *International Journal of Neurosci*, 82(3–4), June 1995, pp. 255–268.

This article reports on the cases of four medicated Parkinsonian patients who experienced reversal of visuospatial impairments as measured by the Clock Drawing Test following treatment with externally applied weak electromagnetic fields of picotesla-range intensity.

R. Sandyk & K. Derpapas, "The Effects of External picoTesla Range Magnetic Fields on the EEG in Parkinson's Disease," *International Journal of Neurosci,* 70(1–2), May 1993, pp. 85–96.

This article reports on the case of a 68-year-old male patient suffering from Parkinson's disease over a period of 7 years. The patient had experienced little relief from traditional medical therapy. Treatment with external application of picotesla-range magnetic fields led to quick improvements with respect to tremor and foot dystonia, gait, postural reflexes, mood, anxiety, and cognitive and autonomic functions.

R. Sandyk & K. Derpapas, "Further Observations on the Unique Efficacy of PicoTesla Range Magnetic Fields in Parkinson's Disease," *International Journal of Neurosci,* 69(1–4), March–April 1993, pp. 67–83.

This article reports on the cases of four Parkinsonian patients who exhibited significant improvements in motor symptoms following treatment with externally applied magnetic fields of picotesla-range intensity.

R. Sandyk & R.P. Iacono, "Rapid Improvement of Visuoperceptive Functions by picoTesla Range Magnetic Fields in Patients with Parkinson's Disease," *International Journal of Neurosci,* 70(3–4), June 1993, pp. 233–254.

This article reports on two cases of fully medicated Parkinson's patients who experienced enhanced visuoperceptive functions as measured by numerous drawing tests following extracranial treatment with picotesla-range magnetic fields.

R. Sandyk, "The Effects of PicoTesla Range Magnetic Fields on Perceptual Organization and Visual Memory in Parkinsonism," *International Journal of Neurosci*, 73(3–4), December 1993, pp. 207–219.

This article reports on the case of a 69-year-old Parkinsonian patient on full medication who experienced a marked improvement on several different drawing tests following 30 minutes of treatment with picotesla-range magnetic fields.

R. Sandyk, et al., "Magnetic Fields in the Treatment of Parkinson's Disease," *International Journal of Neurosci*, 63(1–2), March 1992, pp. 141–150.

This article reports on the case of a Parkinson's patient suffering from severe movement problems who received treatment with external artificial weak magnetic fields with a frequency of 2 Hz and intensity of 7.5 picotesla over a period of 6 minutes. Results showed a significant attenuation in disability and near total reversal of the symptoms lasting approximately 72 hours. The patient then applied equivalent magnetic fields on a daily basis at home. Sustained improvement was seen throughout an observation of one month.

R. Sandyk, "Weak Magnetic Fields in the Treatment of Parkinson's Disease with the "On-off" Phenomenon," *International Journal of Neurosci*, 66(1–2), September 1992, pp. 97–106.

This article reports on the case of a 67-year-old male patient suffering from Parkinson's disease and levodopa-related motor fluctuations. Treatment with the application of external weak magnetic fields led to improvements in general Parkinsonian symptoms along with the amelioration of "on-off" symptoms.

PERIPHERAL NEURITIS

O. Vassilenko and N.F. Vassilenko, "Use of Extremely High Frequency Electromagnetic Radiation for Treating Peripheral Neuritis," Second World Congress for Electricity and Magnetism in Biology and Medicine, 8–13 June 1997, Bologna, Italy.

In this study, patients suffering from peripheral neuritis were exposed to high-frequency electromagnetic radiation on acupuncture points. EMR was generated by Electronica-EnF, Aria, and Porog devices with tunable frequencies ranging between 53 and 78 GHz. Treatments were daily and lasted 25 minutes. Results showed full restoration of nerve function in 87 percent of patients.

PNEUMONIA

E.A. Gaidashev, et al., "An Evaluation of the Effect of Magnetic-laser Therapy on External Respiratory Function in Complicated Forms of Acute Pneumonia in Children," *Vopr Kurortol Fizioter Lech Fiz Kult,* (3), May–June 1995, pp. 12–14.

Results of this study showed that magnetic laser therapy decreased the severity of acute respiratory insufficiency and treatment course, and prevented destructive complications in children with infiltrative acute destructive pneumonia between the ages of 1 and 12 years.

POST-HERPETIC NEURALGIA

C. Kusaka, et al., "Pulse Magnetic Treatment and Whole-Body, Alternating Current Magnetic Treatment for Post-Herpetic Neuralgia," *Journal of Japanese Biomagnetism Bioelectromagnetics Society*, 8(2), 1995, pp. 29–38.

This study found both pulsed magnetic field treatment (20–30 minutes per day) and whole body alternating current magnetic field treatment (30 minutes per day) to be effective therapies for post–herpetic neuralgia in older patients. Pulsed magnetic field treatment consisted of 0.6-T (6-kG) samarium/cobalt magnets surrounded by spiral coils generating a maximum 0.1-T pulse. Pads were pasted on the sensory areas innervated by the dorsal root of the spinal cord where there was scar-association pain or paresthesia. Stimuli were delivered at 280 V and 8 Hz. Alternating current magnetic field treatment involved a treatment bed consisting of 19 electrodes containing paired coils and with a maximum magnetic flux density around the electrodes of 0.08 T.

J.W. Simmons, "Treatment of Failed Posterior Lumbar Interbody Fusion (PLIF) of the Spine with Pulsing Electromagnetic Fields," *Clin Orthop*, (193), March 1985, pp. 127–132.

P. Navratil, et al., "Pulsed Magnetic Field in Therapy of Prostatodynias. A Pilot Study," Bioelectromagnetics Society, 16th Annual Meeting, 12–17 June 1994, Copenhagen, Denmark, pp. 1994.

PSEUDOARTHROSIS

J.S. Kort, et al., "Congenital Pseudoarthrosis of the Tibia: Treatment with Pulsing Electromagnetic Fields," *Clin Orthop*, (165), May 1982, pp. 124–137.

In this study, 92 congenital pseudoarthrosis patients received treatment with pulsing electromagnetic fields. Results indicated a 76 percent rate of lesion recovery.

C.A. Bassett, et al., "Congenital 'Pseudarthroses' of the Tibia: Treatment with Pulsing Electromagnetic Fields," *Clin Orthop*, (154), January–February 1981, pp. 136–148.

In this study, 34 patients with congenital pseudoarthrosis-associated infantile nonunions received treatment with pulsing electromagnetic fields. Results indicated that 50 percent experienced full healing, 21 percent experienced healing with need for protections, and 29 percent experienced failure. The majority of failures were among men with a history of early fracture. Following the demonstration of coil effects, the PEMF treatment was combined with surgical realignment, immobilization, and grafting.

C.A. Bassett, et al., "A Non-operative Salvage of Surgically-resistant Pseudarthroses and Non-unions by Pulsing Electromagnetic Fields. A Preliminary Report," *Clin Orthop*, (124), May 1977, pp. 128–143.

In this study, 29 congenital pseudoarthrosis patients received extremely low frequency pulsing electromagnetic fields. Results: Over 70 percent experienced full healing, 21 percent experienced healing with need for protections, and 29 percent experienced failure. The majority of failures were among men with a history of early fracture.

F. Lechner, et al., "Treatment of Infected Pseudoarthroses with Electrodynamic Field Therapy," *Fortschr Med*, 97(20), May 24, 1979, pp. 943–949.

In this article, the authors report on their own clinical use of electrodynamic field therapy in the treatment of 271 pseudoarthrosis patients over a period of 8 years. They report bone healing in 92 percent of such cases.

C.A. Bassett & M. Schink-Ascani, "Long-term Pulsed Electromagnetic Field (PEMF) Results in Congenital Pseudoarthrosis," *Calcif Tissue Int*, 49(3), September 1991, pp. 216–220.

This study examined the effects of pulsed electromagnetic fields on 91 patients with congenital pseudoarthrosis of the tibia. Results showed an overall success rate of 72 percent.

M.L. Sutcliffe & A.A. Goldberg, "The Treatment of Congenital Pseudoarthrosis of the Tibia with Pusling Electromagnetic Fields: A Survey of 52 Cases," *Clinical Orthop*, (166), 1982, pp. 45–57.

Results of this study indicated that treatment with pulsed electromagnetic fields had beneficial effects in children suffering from congenital pseudoarthrosis.

J.S. Kort & C.A.L. Bassett, "Role of Electricity in the Treatment of Congenital Pseudoarthrosis of the Tibia," *Reconstr Surg Traumatol*, 19, 1985, pp. 140–146.

Results of this study indicated that pulsed electromagnetic fields (72 Hz) can be an effective therapy for patients suffering from lesions associated with congenital pseudoarthroses when treatment is combined with appropriate orthopedic management.

PSYCHIATRIC DISORDERS

T. Zyss, "Deep Magnetic Brain Stimulation—The End of Psychiatric Electroshock Therapy?" *Medical Hypotheses*, 43(2), 1994, pp. 69–74.

Noting the well-established dangers associated with electroconvulsive therapy, the author, in this theoretical article, argues that transcranial magnetic stimulation should be looked at as an alternative psychiatric treatment. The author asserts that TMS has several advantages over ECT in that it is painless, noninvasive, and more effective on deep structures of the brain.

RESPIRATORY PROBLEMS

G.A. Mozhaev & IIu Tikhonovskii, "The Prevention and Treatment of Suppurative-inflammatory Complications in the Bronchopulmonary System During Prolonged Artificial Ventilation," *Anesteziol Reanimatol,* (4), July–August 1002, pp. 47–51.

Results of this study showed that the use of low-frequency magnetic fields helped to prevent and treat critically ill patients suffering from pyoinflammatory bronchopulmonary complications, and to prevent such complications as well.

R. Sandyk & K. Derpapas, "Successful Treatment of Respiratory Dyskinesia with picoTesla Range Magnetic Fields," *International Journal of Neurosci,* 75(1–2), March 1994, pp. 91–102.

This article reports on the case of a schizophrenic patient suffering from respiratory difficulties associated with neuroleptic withdrawal. Treatment using external application of picotesla-range magnetic fields quickly attenuated the severity of such problems.

SEXUAL DISORDERS

I.I. Gorpinchenko, "The Use of Magnetic Devices in Treating Sexual Disorders in Men," *Lik Sprava,* (3-4), March–April 1995, pp. 95–97.

Results of this placebo-controlled study showed that magnetotherapy exhibited beneficial effects with respect to cavernous blood flow in male patients suffering from sexual problems.

I.V. Karpukhin & V.A. Bogomol'nii, "Local Vacuum-Magnetotherapy of Impotency Patients," *Vopr Kurortol Lech Fiz Kult,* (2), 1996, pp. 38–40.

This study examined the effects of a combination pulsing magnetic field (PMF)/vacuum therapy in the treatment of impotence. Vacuum therapy consisted of the penis being placed into a hermetic cylinder with a negative pressure of 180–260 mmHg for 10–12 minutes per exposure for a total of 12–15 exposures. PMF therapy consisted of the same length and number of exposures, with 6 Hz, 30 mT being applied to the penile area at the same time as vacuum therapy. Results showed that, following the combination therapy, sexual function was restored in about 71 percent of patients, was improved in 17 percent, and did not change in 17 percent. For those patients receiving vacuum therapy only, the numbers were 51, 24, and 24 percent, respectively.

I.I. Gorpinchenko, "The Use of Magnetic Devices in Treating Sexual Disorders in Men," *Lik Sprava,* (3–4), 1995, pp. 95–97.

This double-blind, placebo-controlled study examined the effects of weak magnetic fields in men suffering from various sexual disorders, including decreased erection and premature ejaculation. The three different magnetic stimulators used included the "Biopotenzor," "Eros," and "Bioskan-1" devices. All patients wore one of the three devices for a 3-week period. Results showed full restoration of sexual function in 38 percent of patients in the Biopotenzor group, 31 percent in the Eros group, 36 percent in the Bioskan-1 group, and in just 15 percent of the controls. Improvements in sexual function were seen among 42 percent, 39 percent, 47 percent, and 18 percent, respectively.

T.U. Gorgiladze & B.M. Kogan, "A New Method of Treatment of a Dry Kerato-Conjunctivitis in Sjogren's Syndrome," *Oftalmol Zh,* (1), 1996, pp. 38–40.

SLEEP DISORDERS

R. Hajdukovic, et al., "Effects of Low Energy Emission Therapy (LEET) on Sleep Structure," First World Congress for Electricity and Magnetism in Biology and Medicine, 14–19 June 1992, Lake Buena Vista, FL, p. 92.

Results of this double-blind, placebo-controlled study indicated that low-energy-emission therapy significantly improved sleeping patterns among patients suffering from chronic psychophysiological insomnia. Therapy was administered 3 times per week, always in late afternoon and for 20 minutes, over a period of 4 weeks.

M. Erman, et al., "Low-Energy Emission Therapy (LEET) Treatment for Insomnia," Bioelectromagnetics Society, 13th Annual Meeting, 23–27 June 1991, Salt Lake City, UT, p. 69.

This double-blind, placebo-controlled study examined the effects of low-energy-emission therapy (27 MHz amplitude-modulated electromagnetic fields) in patients suffering from insomnia. Treatment consisted of 3 exposures per week over a 4-week period. Results showed significant increases in total sleep time among patients in the treatment group relative to controls.

C. Guilleminault & B. Pasche, "Clinical Effects of Low Energy Emission Therapy," Bioelectromagnetics Society, 15th Annual Meeting, 13–17 June 1993, Los Angeles, CA, p. 84.

This review article notes that studies have found low-energy-emission therapy to be effective in the treatment of chronic insomnia, and suggests that it may also be of value for patients suffering from generalized anxiety disorders.

SPINAL CORD INJURY

E.V. Tkach, et al., "Characteristics of the Effect of a Constant Electromagnetic Field on Reparative Processes in Spinal Cord Injuries," *Zh Nevropatol Psikhiatr*, 89(5), 1989, pp. 41–44.

Results of this study found that exposure to constant magnetic fields improved healing in rats with experimentally induced spinal cord injury, and in human patients suffering from spinal cord trauma as well.

M.K. Sheriff, et al., "Neuromodulation of Detrusor Hyperreflexia Functional Magnetic Stimulation of the Sacral

Roots," *British Journal of Urology*, 78(1), July 1996, pp. 39–46.

This study examined the effects of functional magnetic stimulation used to treat spinal cord injury in seven male patients. Results showed the treatment to be an effective noninvasive approach.

STROKE

L.L. Orlov, et al., "Running Pulse Magnetic Field in Treating Stenocardia," *Biofizika*, 41(4), 1996, pp. 949–952.

F.E. Gorbunov, et al., "The Effect of Combined Transcerebral Magnetic and Electric Impulse Therapy on the Cerebral and Central Hemodynamic Status of Stroke Patients in the Early Rehabilitation Period," *Vopr Kurortol Fizioter Lech Fiz Kult*, (3), May–June 1996, pp. 21–24.

Results of this study demonstrated that treatment with sinusoidal modulated currents coupled with transcerebral magnetic fields proved more effective than either therapy on its own in the treatment of stroke patients during the period of early rehabilitation.

G. Grant, et al., "Protection Against Focal Cerebral Ischemia Following Exposure to a Pulsed Electromagnetic Field," *Bioelectromagnetics*, 15(3), 1994, pp. 205–216.

This study found that exposure to pulsed electromagnetic fields following focal cerebral ischemia provided significant protection against neuronal damage in rabbits.

N.Y. Gilinskaia, "Magnetic Fields in Treatment of Vascular Diseases of the Brain," *Magnitologiia*, 1, 1991, pp. 13–17.

Results of this study pointed to the efficacy of magnetic field therapy in the treatment of patients suffering from a variety of conditions associated with different brain vascular diseases.

SYNOVITIS

A. Weinberger, et al., "Treatment of Experimental Inflammatory Synovitis with Continuous Magnetic Field," *Isr Journal of Med Sci*, 32(12), December 1996, pp. 1197–1201.

This study examined the effects of magnetic fields on synovitis in rats. Results showed that the placement of a 3800-gauss magnet on the bottom of the cage significantly suppressed inflammation associated with the condition, relative to controls.

TENDONITIS

A. Binder, et al., "Pulsed Electromagnetic Field Therapy of Persistent Rotator Cuff Tendinitis. A Double-blind Controlled Assessment," *Lancet*, 1(8379), March 31, 1984, pp. 695–698.

Results of this double-blind, placebo-controlled study indicated that pulsed electromagnetic field therapy exhibited significant beneficial effects in the treatment of patients suffering from persistent rotator cuff tendonitis.

TOURETTE'S SYNDROME

R. Sandyk, "Improvement of Right Hemispheric Functions in a Child with Gilles de la Tourette's Syndrome by Weak Electromagnetic Fields," *International Journal of Neurosci,* 81(3-4), April 1995, pp. 199–213.

This article reports on the case of a 6-year-old boy suffering from Tourette's syndrome who experienced improvements in visuoconstructional and visuomotor skills, along with more general symptomatic improvements, following the extracranial application of electromagnetic fields in the picotesla range of intensity.

TUBERCULOSIS

A. Khomenko, et al., "Use of Millimeter-Range Electromagnetic Radiation in Complex Therapy for Pulmonary Tuberculosis," *Millimetrovie Volni v Biologii I Meditcine,* (3), 1994, pp. 53–61.

This study examined the efficacy of millimeter waves combined with conventional drug treatment in patients suffering from tuberculosis. MW therapy consisted of 10 exposures of the thymus area for 60 minutes per day using a "Yavor" apparatus (6.4 or 7.1 mm wavelength). Controls received drug treatment only. Results indicated that while MW/drug therapy had no effect on the clearance of the tuberculosis bacteria, it did facilitate clinical recovery faster than drug therapy alone.

T.V. Kalinina & V.D. Churaev, "Expense with the Use of the EHF-Therapy at Ryasan' Regional Clinical TB Dispensary," *Millimetrovie Volni v Biologii i Meditcine*, (4), 1994, pp. 52–53.

This study examined the effects of extremely high frequency therapy as administered via a "Yav'-1-7,1" apparatus (7.1 mm wavelength) on tuberculosis patients. Results showed a 25-percent improvement in patients receiving the therapy as a pathogenic treatment. A 72 percent improvement rate was seen among patients who received the therapy as treatment for concurrent diseases.

A.S. Solov'ena, et al., "Use of Constant Magnetic Field for Increasing the Effectiveness of Chemotherapy in Patients with Pulmonary Tuberculosis," *Probl Tuberk*, 8, 1987, pp. 53–56.

This controlled study examined the effects of constant elastic electromagnetic fields (40 mT) in patients suffering from pulmonary tuberculosis. Therapy consisted of 30–45 minute daily application of either a single magnet or a pair of magnets placed on the chest at an area high in skin temperature over a 1–3-month period. When coupled with conventional treatments, one third of patients receiving the constant electromagnetic fields experienced healing of tubercular cavities.

By contrast, only one fifth of patients receiving conventional treatment alone experienced such effects. One month into combination treatment, there was no evidence of mycobacterium tuberculosis in the sputum in half the patients relative to only one third of controls.

ULCERS (GASTRIC AND DUODENAL)

A.V. Alekseenko, et al., "Use of Magnetic Therapy Combined with Galvanization and Tissue Electrophoresis in the Treatment of Trophic Ulcers," Klin Khir, 46(7–8), 1993, p. 31–34.

A. Sieron, et al., "Use of Magnetic Field in Treatment of Trophic Leg Ulcers," Pol Tyg Lek, 46(37–39), September 1991, p. 717–719.

Tiu Kravtsova, et al., "The Use of Magnetic Puncture in Patients with Duodenal Peptic Ulcer," *Vopr Kurortol Fizioter Lech Fiz Kult*, (1), January–February 1994, pp. 22–24.

J. Carion, et al., "New Therapeutic Measures for the Treatment of Ulcers," *Phlebologie*, 31(4), October–December 1978, pp. 339–342.

M.V. Poslavskii, et al., "Treatment of Peptic Ulcer Electromagnetic Irradiation of the Millimetric Range," *Sov Med*, (1), 1989, pp. 29–31.

Results of this study showed that the administration of millimetric electromagnetic waves helped to normalize blood properties, subsequently improving the effectiveness of more conventional gastric and duodenal ulcer treatment.

I.G. Sukhotnik, "Comparitive Effectiveness of Using Constant and Alternating Magnetic Fields in the Treatment of Trophic Ulcers," Vest Khir, 144(6), 1990, p. 123–124.

S. Comorosan, et al., "The Effect of Diapulse Therapy on the Healing of Decubitus Ulcer," Romanian Journal of Physiol, 30(1–2), 1993, p. 41–45.

M.V. Poslavsky, et al., "Experience with Application of Millimeter-Range Radiation for Treatment and Prophylaxis of Stomach and Duodenal Ulcer," *Vopr Kurortol Fizioter Lech Fiz Kult,* (4), 1989, pp. 31–36.

This study examined the effects of millimeter wave (MW) therapy in 317 patients suffering from duodenal and gastric ulcers. MW therapy consisted of 30 minutes per day exposure of the epigastric area ("Yav'-1" apparatus, 10 mW/cm2, 5.6-mm wavelength) until complete ulcer cicatrization was achieved. Results showed a 95 percent rate of ulcer cicatrization in patients receiving the treatment compared to a 78 percent rate in controls. One-year follow-up showed a 54 percent ulcer recurrence rate in MW-treated patients, which was markedly less than the rate for controls.

F.V. Galimzianov, "Laser and Electromagnetolaser Therapy for Trophic Ulcers of the Lower Extremities in Chronic Venous Insufficiency," Vestn Khir Im I I Grek, 152(5–6), 1994, p. 70–72.

M.V. Teppone, et al., "Extremely-High Frequency Therapy of Duodenal Ulcer," *Klin Med*, 69(10), 1991, pp. 74–77.

This controlled study found extremely high frequency therapy to be an effective treatment in patients suffering from duodenal ulcers. Treatment consisted of 5–10 exposures, lasting 20–30 minutes, and making use of the G4-142 apparatus (53.5–70.0 GHz frequency range).

J.E. Kenkre, et al., "A Randomized Controlled Trial of Electromagnetic Therapy in the Primary Care Management of Venous Leg Ulceration," *Family Pract*, 13(3), 1996, pp. 236–241.

S.S. Dudka, et al., "A Comparative Assessment of the Efficacy of Drug Therapy and Microwave Resonance Therapy for Ulcerative Disease of the Duodenum," *Fundamental and Applied Aspects of the Use of Millimeter Electromagnetic Radiation in Medicine*. Abstracts of the 1st All-Union Symposium with International Participation, May 10–13, 1989, Kiev, Ukraine, pp. 195–197.

This study compared the effects of traditional drug treatment (TDT) to those of microwave resonance therapy (MRT) in patients suffering from duodenal ulcers. Results indicated the mean hospital stay for patients in the TDT group was approximately 22 days. Throughout this period, ulcers healed in 38 percent of patients, were reduced in 17 percent, showed no change in 43 percent, and increased in 2 percent. No pain relief was seen in 32 percent. By contrast, mean discharge time for patients in the MRT group was approximately 12 days. Pain was generally stopped in 3–6 days. Complete healing occurred in 81 percent, a decrease was seen in 16 percent, and ulcer size did not change in just 3 percent. Remission occurred in 98 percent of such patients.

V.A. Kutzenok, "Microwave Resonance Therapy of Stomach and Duodenal Ulcers," *Fundamental and Applied Aspects of the Use of Millimeter Electromagnetic Radiation in Medicine.* Abstracts of the 1st All-Union Symposium with International Participation, May 10-13, 1989, Kiev, Ukraine, pp. 192–193.

In this study, microwave resonance therapy (MRT) was administered to 2642 patients suffering from duodenal ulcers and to 78 with gastric ulcers. Treatment involved the use of a G4-142 device (53.6–78.3 GHz, less than 2 mW/cm2 incident power) as well as "Electronika-KVCh" and "Porog-1" devices. Patients received 6–12 daily exposures of between 20 and 25 minutes. Results showed a total ulcer cicatrization in 80 percent of patients, and arrested pain syndrome in almost 100 percent.

T. Kravtzova, et al., "Efficacy of Magnetic Puncture Treatment of Patients with Duodenal Ulcers," *Doktor Lending,* 4(13), 1996, p. 22-24.

ULCERS (TROPHIC)

A.V. Alekseenko, et al., "Use of Magnetic Therapy Combined with Galvanization and Tissue Electrophoresis in the Treatment of Trophic Ulcers," *Klin Khir,* (7–8), 1993, pp. 31–34.

This study examined the use of magnetotherapy coupled with galvanization and intratissue electrophoresis in 86 patients suffering from trophic ulcers. A "Potok-1" apparatus with a density of current equal to 0.05-0.1 mA/cm2 was used to create an electrical field. The "MAG-30" apparatus for low-frequency magnetotherapy with induction of 30 mT and area of exposure of 20 cm2 was applied to a trophic ulcer site at the same time. Results led the authors to conclude that magnetogalvanotherapy is the recommended treatment for trophic ulcers of the lower extremities.

A. Sieron, et al., "Use of Magnetic Field in Treatment of Trophic Leg Ulcers," *Pol Tyg Lek*, 46(37–39), September 1991, pp. 717–719.

This review article discusses the theoretical and clinical applications of magnetic field therapy in the treatment of trophic ulcers of the lower limbs.

I.G. Sukhotnik, "Comparative Effectiveness of Using Constant and Alternating Magnetic Fields in the Treatment of Trophic Ulcers," *Vest Khir*, 144(6), 1990, pp. 123–124.

This study looked at the effects of conventional trophic ulcer treatment alone and in combination with alternating magnetic field (AMF) or constant magnetic field (CMF) exposures in a group of patients suffering from various types of trophic ulcers of the lower limbs. Results showed an average hospital stay of 31 days in the CMF group and 27 days in the AMF group, compared to 40 days among controls. Based on these and related findings, the authors suggest combination AMF therapy to be most effective.

S. Comorosan, et al., "The Effect of Diapulse Therapy on the Healing of Decubitus Ulcer," *Romanian Journal of Physiol,* 30(1–2), 1993, pp. 41–45.

This placebo-controlled study examined the effects of pulsed electromagnetic fields in the treatment of decubitus ulcers in hospitalized elderly patients with stage II and III pressure ulcers. Patients received daily PEMF stimulation in conjunction with conventional treatment for a period of up to 5 weeks. The findings were that combined PEMF/conventional treatment was superior to conventional treatment and to the placebo received by controls.

F.V. Galimzianov, "Laser and Electromagnetolaser Therapy for Trophic Ulcers of the Lower Extremities in Chronic Venous Insufficiency," *Vestn Khir Im I I Grek,* 152(5–6), 1994, pp. 70–72.

Results of this study found that the daily use of electromagnetolaser therapy decreased mean healing time in patients suffering from lower extremity trophic ulcers to approximately 18 days, compared with approximately 26 days in patients receiving laser therapy alone.

C.A. Salzberg, et al., "The Effects of Non-Thermal Pulsed Electromagnetic Energy on Wound Healing of Pressure Ulcers in Spinal Cord-Injured Patients: A Randomized, Double-Blind Study," *Wounds: A Compendium of Clinical Research and Practice,* 7(1), 1995, pp. 11–16.

This double-blind, placebo-controlled study found that treatment with nonthermal pulsed electromagnetic energy

(PEMET) accelerated would healing in spinal cord injury patients suffering from stage II and III pressure ulcers. PEMET treatment consisted of pulsed 27.12-MHz energy produced via a Diapulse device. Energy was delivered by the use of a treatment head placed in wound dressings for 30-minute periods twice a day for 12 weeks or until sores healed.

M. Jeran, et al., "PEMF Stimulation of Skin Ulcers of Venous Origin in Humans: Preliminary Report of a Double-Blind Study," *Journal of Bioelectr,* 6(2), 1987, pp. 181–188.

This double-blind, placebo-controlled study examined the effects of pulsed electromagnetic fields (75 Hz, 2.7 mT) applied 4 hours per day for a maximum of 3 months coupled with conventional therapies in patients suffering from trophic lesions. Results showed the treatment to have positive effects, but only on small lesions.

URINARY PROBLEMS

M.J. Stiller, et al., "A Portable Pulsed Electromagnetic Field (PEMF) Device to Enhance Healing of Recalcitrant Venous Ulcers: A Double-Blind, Placebo-Controlled Clinical Trial," *British Journal of Dermatology,* 127(2), 1992, pp. 146–154.

O.B. Loran, et al., "Magnetic-laser Therapy in Inflammatory and Post-traumatic Lesions of the Urinary System," *Urol Nefrol* (Mosk), (5), September–October 1996, pp. 10–14.

In this article, the authors report on their successful use of magnetic-laser therapy in inflammations of the urinary system in a urological clinic setting.

V.P. Avdoshin, et al., "Assessment of Magnetolaser Therapy in Comparison with Other Methods of Treatment of Patients with Urolithiasis," *Fiz Med*, 4(1–2), 1994, pp. 102–103.

Results of this study showed magnetolaser therapy to be effective in the treatment of patients suffering from urolithiasis (stone formation). Magnetolaser therapy involved the use of a Milita device with a 35-mT magnetic field.

M. Karczewska, "Use of Magnetic Therapy for Treatment of Early Symptoms of Vascular-type Vibration Syndrome in Forestry Workers," *Med Pr*, 47(4), 1996, 373–381.

A.E. Mal'tsev, "The Magnetic Amplipulse Therapy of Vestibular Dysfunctions of Vascular Origin Using the Sedaton Apparatus," *Vopr Kurortol Fizioter Lech Fiz Kult*, (1), January–February 1994, pp. 16–19.

WOUND HEALING

S. Saha, et al., "Effect of Electrical Stimulation of Wound Healing: A Review," Second World Congress for Electricity and Magnetism in Biology and Medicine, 8–13 June 1997, Bologna, Italy.

D. Man, et al., "Effect of Permanent Magnetic Field on Postoperative Pain and Wound Healing in Plastic Surgery,"

Second World Congress for Electricity and Magnetism in Biology and Medicine, 8–13 June 1997, Bologna, Italy.

This study examined the effects of static magnetic fields on postoperative wounds in 21 patients undergoing plastic surgery. Magnetic patches ranging in thickness from 1 to 6 mm, and 2450 to 3950 G field strength were administered over the area of operation for a total of 48 hours. Thirteen patients received the magnets after pain or edema had appeared and 8 received them prophylactically. Results showed a decrease in pain, edema, and coloration in approximately 60 percent of patients. Such symptoms disappeared entirely in 75 percent.

B. Vukovic-Jankovic, et al., "Peripheral Nerve Regeneration Stimulated by Pulsating Electromagnetic (PEMF) Field and Laser," Second World Congress for Electricity and Magnetism in Biology and Medicine, 8–13 June 1997, Bologna, Italy.

Results of this study indicated that treatment with pulsating electromagnetic field either alone or in combination with laser therapy exhibited healing effects with respect to peripheral nerve lesions and general wound healing relative to controls.

M.J. McLean, et al., "Treatment of Wrist Pain in the Work Place with a Static Magnetic Device—Interim Report of a Clinical Trial," Second World Congress for Electricity and Magnetism in Biology and Medicine, June 8–13, Bologna, Italy.

This double-blind, placebo-controlled study examined the effects of a magnetic treatment device taped over the carpal tunnel against wrist pain sustained at work among a group of turkey plant employees. Results showed that the device was effective in alleviating such pain and that it was free of side effects.

O. Patino, et al., "Pulsed Electromagnetic Fields in Experimental Cutaneous Wound Healing in Rats," *Journal of Burn Care Rehabil,* 17(6 PT 1), 1996, pp. 528–531.

Results of this controlled study showed that low-frequency pulsed electromagnetic fields produced significant beneficial cutaneous wound healing effects in rats.

C.A. Salzberg, et al., "The Effects of Non-Thermal Pulsed Electromagnetic Energy on Wound Healing of Pressure Ulcers in Spinal Cord-Injured Patients: A Randomized, Double-Blind Study," *Ostomy Wound Manage,* 41(3), 1995, pp. 42–51.

This double-blind, placebo-controlled study found that treatment with nonthermal pulsed radio frequency energy accelerated wound healing in spinal cord injury patients suffering from Stage II and III pressure ulcers. RF treatment consisted of pulsed 27.12-MHz energy produced via a Diapulse device, with energy delivered via a treatment head placed in wound dressings for 30-minute periods twice a day for 12 weeks or until sores healed.

G.C. Coats, "Pulsed Electromagnetic (Short-Wave) Energy Therapy," *British Journal of Sports Medicine,* 23(4), 1989, pp. 213–216.

After a discussion of the mechanics involved in the use of pulsed electromagnetic energy in the treatment of disease, the author discusses findings from recent studies pointing to the therapy's effectiveness with respect to the treatment of acute soft-tissue lesions.

N.N. Korpan & T. Saradeth, "Clinical Effects of Continous Microwave for Postoperative Septic Wound Treatment: A Double-Blind Controlled Trial," *American Journal of Surgery*, 170(3), 1995, pp. 271–276.

Results of this placebo-controlled study indicated that low-intensity continuous microwave radiation administered over a period of 7 days was effective in treating postoperative purulent wounds associated with abdominal surgery.

N. Bairamov, et al., "Magnetolaser Therapy in Complex Treatment of Gunshot Wounds," All-Union Symposium: Laser and Magnetic Therapy in Experimental and Clinical Studies, 16–18 June 1993, Obnisk, Kaluga Region, Russia, pp. 184–185.

Results of this study showed that combined magneto/laser therapy reduced inflammation and wound suppuration, and enhanced tissue healing significantly in patients suffering from gunshot wounds relative to conventional treatment only.

B.F. Sisken & J. Walker, "Therapeutic Aspects of Electro-magnetic Fields for Soft-Tissue Healing," in M. Blank, (ed.), *Electromagnetic Fields: Biological Interactions and Mech-*

anisms, Washington, D.C.: American Chemical Society, 1995, pp. 277–285.

Noting that pulsed electromagnetic fields have been used in bone healing for more than 20 years, this review article cites recent results from both animal and human studies pointing to the efficacy of PEMF in the treatment of soft-tissue injuries as well.

R.H.C. Bentall & H.B. Eckstein, "A Trial Involving the Use of Pulsed Electro-Magnetic Therapy on Children Undergoing Orchidopexy," *Z. Kinderchir,* 17(4), 1975, pp. 380–389.

This double-blind study examined the effects of postoperative nonthermal pulsed high-frequency electromagnetic fields on edema formation and bruise healing in boys undergoing orchidopexy. Treatment involved exposure 3 times daily for the first 4 days following surgery. Significant effects with respect to rate of bruise resolution were reported in patients receiving the treatment relative to controls.

L.S. Teren'eva, et al., "Treatment of Chronic Productive Inflammation of Orbital Tissues with a Pulsed Electromagnetic Field," *Oftalmol Zh,* 1, 1996, pp. 1–5.

This controlled study examined the effects of pulsed electromagnetic fields in patients suffering from chronic productive inflammation or orbital tissue. PEMF treatment consisted of 7–10 minute daily exposures over a period of 10 days. Controls received conventional treatment only. Both groups showed good improvement, but patients treated with the PEMFs recovered significantly faster than did controls.

Resources

Dr. William Pawluk can be reached at @Compuserve.com or at (773) 388-2961.

Where to Get Magnetic Products

Albert Roy Davis Research Labs
Walter C. Rawls (for information and books)
P.O. Box 655
Green Cove Springs, FL 32043
904-264-8564

American Health Service
694 S. Waukegan Rd., Dept. F
Lake Forest, IL 60045
1-800-544-7521

Ameriflex, Inc.
232 NE Lincoln St., Suite G

Hillsboro, OR 97124
503-640-0810
Fax: 503-640-0517

BEMI
Dr. John Zimmerman
2490 W. Moana Ln.
Reno, NV 89509
702-827-9099
   Dr. Zimmerman provides a comprehensive information package on over two dozen companies selling therapeutic magnetic products, ranging from the two largest, Nikken

and Japan Life, all the way to mom-and-pop operations that sell far less. Some that he recommends highly are Nikken, Magnet Therapy, Inc. (also called Tectonics), and Magnet Relief. The latter is particularly noteworthy for its well-designed magnetic pads. His packet costs $10, which helps to provide support for the Bio-Electro-Magnetics Institute to carry on its research.

Bio-Magnetics
Attn.: Larry Molnar
P.O. Box 223
Bowie, AZ 85605
602-847-2209

Body Magnetics
871 Thrall Avenue
Suffield, CT 06078
203-231-2377

Breakthrough Media, Inc.
5065 SW 153rd Avenue
Beaverton, OR 97007
800-321-5641

The Cutting Edge Catalog
PO Box 5034

South Hampton, NY 11969
800-497-9516

Dendee International
Dennis & Delores Mosher
P.O. Box 106
Clearlake, IA 50428
515-357-7893

Enviro-Tech Products
Dr. William or Katherine
  Philpott
or Len or Joyce Lothrup
17171 SE 29th St.
Choctaw, OK 73020
800-445-1962
405-390-3499
Fax: 405-390-2968

His Way
Magnetic Health Products
Route 30 Mall
Clementon, NJ 08021
800-307-9991

HSW Systems
Russell Hojnowski
P.O. Box 68127
Virginia Beach, VA 23471
800-793-3757
Internet: http://www.soul-
  tions.com

Interceptor Industries
Bio-Magnetic Products
P.O. Box 827
Lake Orion, MI 48361
888-736-8811

Japan Life
(multilevel marketing
    company)
One Executive Drive
Fort Lee, NJ 07024
201-944-7790
Fax: 201-944-5507

LHASA Medical, Inc.
539 Accord Station
Accord, MA 02018-0539
800-722-8775
617-335-6484
Fax: 617-335-6296

Magna-Pak, Inc.
P.O. Box 27106
London, Ontario
Canada N5X 3X5

MagneTherapy Products
4926 Indian Springs Ct.
Plant City, FL 33565
813-757-0508
813-757-6770

MagnetiCo, Inc.
Dr. Dean Bonlie
#107, 5421 11th St N.E.
Calgary, Alberta T2E 6M4
    Canada
800-265-1119
403-730-0883

Magnetic Health Products
5 Burns Street
Byron Bay, 2481 UK
066-857-842 (tel./fax)

Magnetic Therapeutic
    Technology, Inc.
1701 W. Walnut Hills Lane
    #110
Irving, TX 75038
800-371-1113
214-756-6667

Magnetic Wellness Centers
9711 Montgomery Rd.
Cinti, OH 45242
800-484-7964 (code 1956)

Magnet-X Corporation
#8, 2180 Pegasus Way
Calgary, Alberta T2E 8M5
    Canada
800-667-0000
403-291-3090

Mid-American Marketing
PO Box 124
Eaton, OH 45320
800-922-1744
219-749-6666
Fax: 513-456-5424

NeuroMagnetic Systems
William or Leane Roffey-
   Orlando
999 E. Basse Rd., Suite 180
San Antonio, TX 78209
210-824-5352

Nikken, Inc.
(multilevel marketing
   company)
10866 Wilshire Blvd., Suite
   250
Los Angeles, CA 90024
800-669-8859
310-446-4300

Norso Biomagnetics, Inc.
Jim Sauder
4105 Starboard Court
Raleigh, NC 27613
800-480-8601
919-783-5911
919-781-8374

Oriental Medical Supplies, Inc.
1950 Washington Street

Braintree, MA 02184
800-323-1839
617-331-3370
Fax: 617-335-5770

Planetary Herbal Products
Box 7145
Santa Cruz, CA 95061
800-464-1233

Post International
P.O. Box 788
Roy, WA 98580
206-843-1321

PsychoPhysics Labs
Dr. Buryl Payne
4264 Topsail Ct.
Soquel, CA 95073
408-462-1588

Quantum Magnetics
Magnet Relief Products
2602 South Dixie Highway,
   Suite 7
West Palm Beach, FL
   33401
800-525-0644
561-832-9971.

R.D.G. Technologies, Inc.
Bill Roper

913 9th Terrace
Palm Beach Gardens, FL
   33418
407-625-0462

Ruck Enterprises, Inc.
650 West Grand Avenue,
   Unit 110
Elmhurst, Il. 60126
800-366-7825

SBJ Enterprises
4036 W. Grand Blanc Road
   #800
Swartz Creek, MI 48472
810-750-8484

Tengam
Tom Nellessen
4957 Bittrich-Antler Road
Dear Park, WA 99006
509-276-2054

ADDITIONAL READING

The Anatomy of Biomagnetism
By Albert Roy Davis, Ph.D

The Art of Magnetic Healing
By Santwani

Biomagnetic Handbook: A Guide to Medical Magnets: The Energy of Tomorrow
By William H. Philpott, M.D. and Sharon Taplin

The Body Electric: Electromagnetism and The Foundation of Life
By Robert O. Becker, M.D., and Gary Seldon

The Body Magnetic
By Dr. Buryl Payne

The Book of Magnetic Healing & Treatments
By Noel C. Norris

The Cancer Cure that Worked: Fifty Years of Suppression
By Barry Lynes with John Crane

Cross Currents
By Robert O. Becker

Discovery of Magnetic Health: A Health Care Alternative
By George J. Washnis and Richard Z. Hircak

The Electric Wilderness
By Andrew Marino and Joel Ray

Electromagnetic Pollution Solution
By Glen Swartout

Getting Started in Magnetic Healing
By Dr. Buryl Payne

Healing Magnetism
By Heinz Schiegl

Magnet Therapy
By Holger Hannemann

The Magnetic Blueprint of Life
By Albert Roy Davis and Walter C. Rawls, Jr.

The Magnetic Effect
By Albert Roy Davis and Walter C. Rawls, Jr.

Magnetic Field Therapy Handbook
By R. Allen Walls

Magnet Therapy: Balancing Your Body's Energy Flow for Self-Healing
By Holger Hanneman

Magnet Therapy Theory and Practice
By Dr. Neville S. Bengali

Magnetic/Oxygen Answer for Infection and Toxicity
By William H. Philpott, M.D.

Magnetism and its Effect on the Living System
By Albert Roy Davis and Walter C. Rawls, Jr.

Medical Magnets: Nature's Healing Energy
By Barbara Gordon

The Secret of Life: Cosmic Rays and Radiations of Living Beings
By Georges Lakhovsky

Terminal Shock: The Health Hazards of Video Display Terminals
By Bob Dematto

Your Complete Guide to TENS
By Barbara Gordon

Vibrational Medicine: New Choices for Healing Ourselves
By Richard Gerber

The Zapping of America: Microwaves, Their Deadly Risk, and the Coverup
By Paul Brodeur